Fatty Liver Diet Cookbook

200 Liver Friendly Recipes to Reverse Fatty Liver Disease, Lose Weight and Regain Your Health

PETER Nikki

TABLE OF CONTENTS

INTRODUCTION

You can reverse fatty liver disease if you know how!
This book in your hand will help to make reversing fatty liver disease very easy. The original aim of the treatment is to prevent the excess fat buildup which will result in reduction of fat in the weight of the liver. Preventing excess fat buildup can be achieved by changes in your diet, properly managing your weight and taking some exercise. This cookbook in your hand is written to help you to transform your diet. It has over 200 liver friendly recipes with ingredients that will help to nourish the body, prevent fat buildup, lose excess weight and maintain a healthy body.

The liver is one of the most vital organs in our body. It handles critical processes that are indispensable to life and wellbeing. Liver functions is numerous, it includes
1. Storage of nutrients in our body until they are needed for energy
2. Production of bile for easy food digestion
3. Fight infections, by destroying bacteria in our blood
4. Creation and storage of blood clotting agents in our body
 5. Detoxifying the body by removing or changing the work of hormones, chemical, drugs and toxins that is in the body.
6. Storage of vitamins in the body
Fatty liver disease prevents the liver from carrying out all these functions which leads to all kinds of side effects in the body and many other health conditions.
Nonalcoholic fatty liver disease is a situation that allows excess fat buildup in the liver. To have some portion of fat in your liver is normal when it's between 5-10 percent of the liver weight but when the portion of fat is more than that, it's called fatty liver. This excess fat buildup in the liver is usually accompanied by swelling or inflammation of the liver and a reduction in functioning appropriately. If nothing is done on time, it can result to scarring liver damage or even liver failure.
Symptoms of fatty liver disease

Fatty liver disease may occur without any specific symptoms but usually the affected person may have some experience like
-Weight loss
-Tiredness
-Weakness of the body
- Changes in the skin, like yellowing or itching
- Loss of appetite
- Nausea

-Upper right abdominal pain

Fatty liver disease affects about 25 percent of the American population according to research. On the other hand, it is more common among people who have:

- Diabetes
- Have high cholesterol
- Unhealthy diets
-who are obese

If you are experiencing any of the symptoms listed above that means you will need to visit your doctor for testing. The doctor has to carry out some blood tests to check the liver enzymes, imaging of liver and the liver biopsy

Treatment of fatty liver disease

Fatty liver disease does not have any precise medical treatments. It can only respond effectively to changes in diet and a healthy lifestyle with exercise on a regular basis. The recipes in this book will help you to move with no effort from your present diet to healthy foods which are made with liver friendly recipes. The recipes in this book will help you to lose excess fat, reverse fatty liver disease and become healthier. The recipes are very easy and quick to cook and they are so yummy.

It is very important to consult a doctor who specializes in liver disease before embarking on this self healing journey. Even if your test result shows that your liver condition is in order, this diet will still help to protect your liver from any liver disease. The diet will help you to:

- Avoid added sugar in your diet
 -Eat whole grains
-Eat enough vegetable
 -fruits and healthy fats

This diet will help you to eat healthy and stop eating all kinds of unhealthy foods that lead to fat buildup. It will also help to lower cholesterol and control diabetes if you have them

The suggested lifestyles for treating fatty liver or maintaining healthy liver include:

1. Exercising on a regular basis, at least 3-4 time in a week
2. Try to lose weight if you are over weight
3. Quit smoking if you are the type that smoke because fatty liver gets worst with smoking
4. Reduce or avoid taking alcohol
5. Make sure that you get enough sleep and rest every day.

Make use of the recipes in this book, take exercise on a regular basis and make sure you take your medication as prescribed if you have any, with this i am sure your overall health will be in order. I wish all the best!

BREAKFAST RECIPES

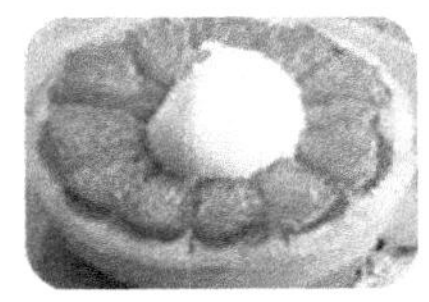

Breakfast Chia Seed Smoothie

This recipe is packed with vitamins and mineral. It's quick and easy to prepare
Total time: 5 minutes
Prep time: 5 minutes
Cook time: 0 minutes
Servings: 4
Ingredients:
2 tbsp. chia seeds
1/2 cup grapefruit juice
1/2 cup frozen raspberries
1/2 cup light coconut milk
1/2 cup pineapple juice
1/2 cup crushed ice
1 tsp. Stevia
Instructions:
1. Combine all the ingredients in a blender bowl and blend until very smooth and creamy.
2. Remove from the blender bowl and serve right away.
Nutrition (per serving): | 102 calories, | protein 1g, | carbohydrate13g s, | fiber 2g, | sugar10.4g, | fat 13g, | sodium 4mg | Potassium: 0mg |

Matcha Waffle

Make this gluten-free recipe with these 9 ingredients. It tastes so good.
Total time: 20 minutes
Prep time: 5 minutes
Cook time: 15 minutes
Servings: 5
Ingredients:
The dry ingredients
2 cups gluten-free flour blend
2 tsp. baking powder
21/2 tsp. matcha powder
1/2 tsp. baking soda

The wet ingredients
1/4 cup honey
2 large eggs
1 teaspoon vanilla extract
11/2 cups sugar almond milk
2 tbsp. melted coconut oil
Instructions:
1. Preheat the waffle maker to medium heat.
2. Combine the dry ingredients in a medium bowl and whisk well.
3. Crack the two eggs in a medium bowl and whisk well, add the rest of the wet ingredients except the coconut oil, mix well.
4. Gradually add the dry ingredients into wet ingredients and mix well.
5. Add the coconut oil and mix until smooth.
6. Place 1/2 cup of the batter into the heated waffle maker, close the lid and cook for 3 minutes.
7. Remove from heat and place in a wire rack and then repeat the process with the remaining batter until no more batter.
8. Top the waffles with maple syrup and whipped cream and enjoy!
Nutrition (per serving): | 292calories, | protein 5g, | carbohydrate 52 g, | fiber 2g, | sugar10.4g, | fat 6g, | sodium 0mg | Potassium: 0mg |

Pumpkin Flax Granola

This recipe is crunchy and satisfying! Serve with smoothie or yogurt.
Total time: 25 minutes
Prep time: 5minutes
Cook time: 19 minutes
Servings: 6
Ingredients:
1 cup pumpkin seeds shelled
3 cups Rolled oats Old fashioned whole grain
1/4 cup flax seeds
1/4 cup honey
1/4 cup maple syrup
1/2 cup sugar-free coconut flakes
1/4 cup olive oil
1/2 tsp. salt
Instructions:
1. Preheat the oven to 325°F
2. Combine the oats, pumpkin seeds, coconut flakes and flax seeds in a large bowl.
3. Combine oil, maple syrup, honey and salt in a microwave safe bowl, stir well and microwave for 30 seconds.

4. Slowly drizzle the liquid mixture into the dry mixture and stir gently until well coated.

5. Prepare a large baking sheet with parchment paper. Pour the mixture in the baking sheet, place in the heated oven and bake for 20 minutes, stir once in the middle of the time.

6. Remove from heat, set aside to cool down before crumbling with your hands and then store in airtight container at room temperature.

7. Serve with smoothie or yogurt of choice, enjoy!

Nutrition (per serving): | 113calories, | protein 2g, | carbohydrate 13 g, | fiber 1g, | sugar 0g, |fat 6g, | sodium 0mg | Potassium: 0mg |

Aprese Avocado Toast

This avocado toast is packed with flavor, so yummy and easy to prepare.

Total time: 20 minutes

Prep time: 10 minutes

Cook time: 10 minutes

Servings: 2

Ingredients:

1 avocado

1/2 lemon juice

2 thick slices sourdough, toasted

1 cup mozzarella balls

1/2 cup halved cherry tomatoes

Flaky sea salt

Balsamic glaze, for drizzling

2 basil leaves, freshly sliced

Salt to taste

Freshly ground black pepper to taste

Instructions:

1. Put the avocado in a large bowl, add the lemon juice and mash well with a fork, season with salt and pepper to taste.

2. Spread mashed avocado and lemon juice mixture on toast and top with mozzarella and cherry tomatoes. Enjoy!

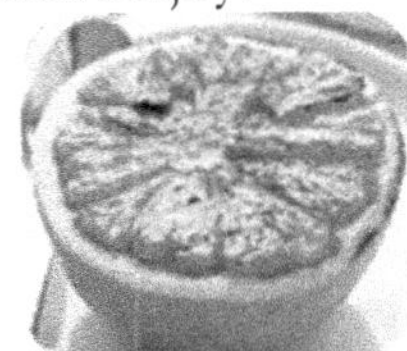

Broiled Grapefruit

This recipe is quick and easy to prepare

Total time: 16 minutes

Prep time: 10 minutes
Cook time: 6 minutes
Servings: 1
Ingredients:
1 grapefruit (cut in half)
1 tsp. honey
1/2 tsp. ground ginger
1/2 Strawberries (finely slice)
Instructions:
1. Prepare your oven rack and set your oven for broiling
2. Place the grapefruit halves on a baking pan.
3. Drizzle honey over the grapefruit halves. Place the slices of strawberries over it and then flip to coat well with honey. Add the ground ginger.
4. Place the baking pan under broiler for 6 minutes or until bubbling and slightly browned. Check often to avoid burning.
5. Remove from heat and serve right away. Enjoy!
Nutrition (per serving): | 59 calories, | protein 1.1g, | carbohydrate 15.2 g, | fiber 2.2g, | sugar 21.5g, | fat 0g, | sodium 101mg | Potassium: 0mg |

Grapefruit Honey Mint Tea

Total time: 16 minutes
Prep time: 10 minutes
Cook time: 6 minutes
Servings: 1
Ingredients:
3/4 cup drinkable waters
2 sprigs of mint
1 grapefruit, juiced.
1 1/2 tsp. Honey
Instructions:
1. Pour the water in a small saucepan, add the sprigs and bring to boil over medium-high heat
2. Reduce the heat low heat and let it simmer for 3 minutes and then gently remove the sprigs of mint from the saucepan.
3. Add the grapefruit juice and honey to the saucepan, taste and adjust taste as needed.
4. Remove from heat and serve. Enjoy!
Nutrition (per serving): | 38 calories, | protein 1g, | carbohydrate 9.8 g, | fiber 1g, | sugar 9g, | fat 0g, | sodium 132mg | Potassium: 0mg |

Low carb Avocado Deviled Eggs

This avocado deviled egg is so yummy!

Total time: 10 minutes
Prep time: 10 minutes
Cook time: 0 minutes
Servings: 6
Ingredients:
6 eggs, hardboiled, cooled and peeled
1/2 cup avocado
1/2 tomato, deseeded and finely diced
2 tsp. red onion, finely minced
Salt and pepper to taste
Instructions:
1. Carefully remove the yolks from the white eggs and place in a bowl
2. Add the guacamole and mash well to combine, season with salt and pepper to taste
3. Add he minced red onion and mix well.
4. Scoop the mixture into the egg white.

Grapefruit Tart with a Coconut Crust

This grapefruit tart is sweet and refreshing
Total time: 4 hour 40 minutes
Prep time: 30 minutes
Cook time: 10 minutes
Servings: 19
Ingredients:
CRUST:
 1 3/4 cup graham cracker crumbs
1/2 cup unsweetened coconut flakes
 1/4 cup granulated sugar
1/3 cup unsalted butter, melted
FILLING:
1 1/2 cups grapefruit juice
3/4 cup sugar
6 tbsp. butter cut in cubes
 3 tbsp. cornstarch
3egg yolks
1/4 teaspoon salt
TOPPING:
1/4 cup toasted coconut flakes
 2 tsp. Chopped dry roasted pistachio nuts
Instructions:
1. Preheat the oven to 400°F and properly coat a rectangular tart pan with nonstick cooking oil.

2. Place the graham cracker crumbs in the bowl of the food processor, add salt and sugar and pulse until well mixed.
3. Gradually add the melted butter on the mixture and continue to pulse until well mixed.
4. Transfer the mixture to a bowl and add the coconut flakes
5. Press into the bottom of coated tart pan and bake until lightly brown, for 7 minutes.
6. Remove from heat and let completely cool down in a rack.
7. Add the cornstarch alongside with the grapefruit and sugar in a saucepan and cook over medium-high heat, cook and stir until mixture is thickened and bubbly.
8. Slowly add 1/2 of the cornstarch mixture to the egg yolks to temper the eggs.
9. Add the eggs mixture back to the saucepan, cook and stir often for about 3 minutes or until thickens
10. Remove the saucepan from heat and add the butter pieces and whisk well until melted.
11. Pour mixture into the crust and smooth the top with spatula. Cover with any plastic wrap pressed against the top of the tart and place in the freezer for 4 hours or overnight.
12. Top with pistachios and coconut flakes and enjoy!
Nutrition (per serving): 290 calories, | protein 1g, | carbohydrate 32.8g, | fiber 2g, | sugar 20g, | fat 15.3g, | sodium 278mg| Potassium: 0mg |

Avocado Egg Boats

This recipe is super creamy and pairs well with crispy bacon and egg. it can serve as a breakfast or snacks.
Total time: 38 minutes
Prep time: 5 minutes
Cook time: 33 minutes
Servings: 4
Ingredients:
2 avocados, halved & pitted
3 slices bacon
4 large eggs
Salt and pepper to taste
Freshly chopped chives, for garnish

Instructions:
1. Preheat the oven to 350°F.
2. Scoop 1 tbsp. worth of avocado out of each half and then reserve for another use.
3. Place in a baking dish. Crack the eggs into a small bowl, one at a time.
4. Place one egg yolk in each avocado half first before adding the egg white to the avocado (don't let it drop aside the avocado)
5. Add salt and pepper to taste and bake for about 25 minutes or until white egg is set. (Cover the baking sheet with foil when the avocado start to brown)
6. In a skillet over medium-high heat, cook the bacon for about 8 minute or until crisp.
7. Remove the bacon from heat and place on a plate lined with a paper towel and cut.
8. To serve, place avocados and bacon on a serving plate, garnish with chives and enjoy.
Nutrition (per serving): 220 calories, |protein 10g, | carbohydrate 6g, | fiber 5g, | sugar 0g, | fat 18g, | sodium 180mg | Potassium: 0mg |

Grapefruit Scones

This grapefruit scone is for your breakfast; enjoy it with a cup of coffee.
Total time: 35 minutes
Prep time: 15 minutes
Cook time: 20 minutes
Servings: 8
Ingredients:
2 cups almond flour blend
1 tbsp. baking powder
2 tbsp. fresh grated grapefruit zest
1 tbsp. almond milk
1/3 cup sugar
1/4 tsp. salt
1/2 cup (1 stick) butter, cut into cubes
3/4 cup fresh squeezed grapefruit juice
ICING
Splash of grapefruit juice
1 cup powdered sugar
Instructions:
1. Preheat the oven to 450°F
2. Combine almond flour, baking powder, salt and sugar in a bowl and whisk gradually to mix until combing.

3. Cut in the butter in a pastry blender and process until crumbly and the size of peas.

4. Add the grapefruit zest and 1/2 of the grapefruit juice to the mixture and process until well combined.

5. Gradually add more grapefruit juice until as you process until dough is moistened.

6. Transfer into a lightly coated cookie sheet and press into 10"circle plate. Cut dough into 8 pieces and separate on a baking sheet to avoid baking into others. Brush the top of the dough with almond milk.

7. Place in the oven and bake until golden brown, for about 20 minutes. Remove from heat and down before frosting.

8. In a mixing bowl, combine grapefruit juice and sugar (add the juice gradually until icing is thin as needed)

Nutrition (per serving): 330 calories, | protein 4g, | carbohydrate 50g|, fiber 1g, | sugar 25g, |fat 13g, | sodium 238mg | Potassium: 0mg |

Healthy Steel Cut Oatmeal

You will surely love this homemade oatmeal, it's so healthy.

Total time: 8 hours 5 minutes

Prep time: 5 minutes

Cook time: 8 hours

Servings: 4

Ingredients:

1 cup steel-cut oats

2 cups skim milk

2 cups water

1/3 cup golden raisins

1/2 tsp. cinnamon

2 tbsp. brown sugar

1/4 tsp. salt

Instructions:

1. In a large crock-pot, combine the skim milk, steel-cut oats, cinnamon, water, golden raisins, brown sugar, and salt and then gently stir well with a spoon until combine.

2. Put on the crock-pot, close the lid and cook until oats is tender, for about 8 hours.

3. Remove from heat and scoop to a serving plate, top with a little skim milk if you want and enjoy

Nutrition (per serving): 176calories, protein 6g, carbohydrate 34 g, fiber 3g, sugar 0g, fat 1g, sodium 0mg | Potassium: 0mg |

Grapefruit Tequila Slammer

This recipe is quick and easy to prepare, it's refreshing and perfect for winter period.
Total time: 5 minutes
Prep time: 5 minutes
Cook time: 0 minutes
Servings: 8
Ingredients:
4 oz. freshly squeezed grapefruit juice plus more for garnish
2 oz. silver tequila
2 oz. lemon lime soda
1/2 cup crushed ice
Instructions:
1. Combine all the ingredients in a glass cup to mix, cover the top of glass with hand and give it a good shake.
2. Serve and enjoy.

Nutrition (per serving): 206 calories, | protein 0g, | carbohydrate 18g, | fiber 0g, sugar 18g, |fat 0g, | sodium 101mg | Potassium: 183mg |

Yummy Grapefruit Sorbet

Total time: 1 hour
Prep time: 15 minutes
Cook time: 0 minutes
Servings: 5
Ingredients:
5 1/2 cups freshly squeezed grapefruit juice
1 tsp. Stevia
Instructions:
1. In a saucepan over medium-high heat, add 1 cup of grapefruit alongside with stevia, whisk and cook for 6 minutes.
2. Remove the saucepan from heat and transfer to a bowl, add the rest of the grapefruit and put in the fridge until chilled.
3. Remove from the fridge and transfer to an ice cream maker and mix according to the directions.
4. pour in a container and put in a freezer for 7 hours or until frozen. Enjoy!

Nutrition (per serving): 109 calories, | protein 1g, | carbohydrate 28.7g, | fiber 1g, sugar 27.7g, |fat 0g, | sodium 0mg | Potassium: 0mg |

Fresh Fruit Salad with Blackberries and Grapefruit

This recipe is loaded with nutrient and taste good.

Total time: 10minutes
Prep time: 10 minutes
Cook time: 0 minutes
Servings: 4

Ingredients:

2 Red Grapefruits – peeled and cut into segment
18 oz. fresh blackberries
5 oz. vanilla yogurt
2 mint leaves finely slice
Pinch flaked sea salt

Instructions:

1. Combine the blackberries and grapefruit in a serving plate and top with slice mint leaves.
2. Add a pinch of sea salt and Greek yogurt and then stir well to mix. Enjoy!

Nutrition (per serving): 139 calories, | protein 5g, | carbohydrate 31g, | fiber 9g, sugar 20g, | fat 1g, | sodium 59mg | Potassium: 0mg |

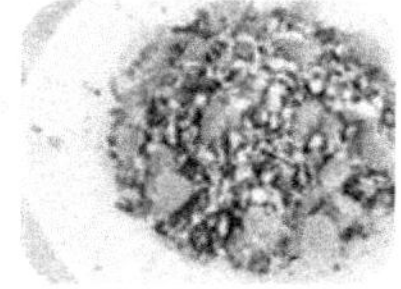

Quinoa and Grapefruit Bowl

This quinoa and grapefruit bowl is nutritious and satisfying, you will love it

Total time: 20minutes
Prep time: 5 minutes
Cook time: 15 minutes
Servings: 1

Ingredients:

1/2 cup quinoas washed and drain
1 cup almond milk
1/2 tsp. cinnamon powder
1/2 grapefruits, peeled and sliced
6 walnuts
1 tbsp. vanilla yogurt

Instructions:

1. Place the washed quinoas in a medium pot alongside with almond milk
2. Add the cinnamon powder to the pot, stir well and cook on a low heat for 15 minutes. Stir every few minutes as you cook.

3. Remove pot from heat when there is no more liquid in the quinoa. Cover the pot set aside
4. To serve, Place quinoa in a serving plate, add walnuts, grapefruit and yogurt, stir well. Enjoy!
Nutrition (per serving): 459 calories, | protein 17g, | carbohydrate 66g, | fiber 32g, sugar 0g, | fat 16g, | sodium 321mg | Potassium: 0mg |

Iced Coffee Protein Shake

This coffee protein shake is so quick and easy to prepare.
Total time: 5 minutes
Prep time: 5 minutes
Cook time: 0 minutes
Servings: 2
Ingredients:
1 1/2 cups ice cubes
1 frozen banana
3/4 cup almond milk
1 tbsp. chocolate protein powder
1 cup coffee, cooled
Instructions:
1. Combine all the ingredients in a blender or food processor and blend until very smooth
2. Transfer to a serving glass cup and enjoy immediately.
Nutrition (per serving): 188 calories, | protein 11g, | carbohydrate 24g, | fiber 3g, sugar 0g, | fat 5g, | sodium 0mg | Potassium: 0mg |

Grapefruit and Strawberry Greyhound Poptail

Total time: 15minutes
Prep time: 5 minutes
Cook time: 1 0 minutes
Servings: 18
Ingredients:
1 Ib. fresh-squeezed grapefruit juice
5 oz. vodka
12 medium strawberries
Instructions:
1. Place the strawberries and the grapefruit juice in the bowl of blender or food processor and process until smooth.
2. Add vodka to the food processor bowl and process for more 30 seconds. Transfer mixture to a popsicles mold.

3. Place a foil on top of the Popsicle and cut a small hole in the center of each well. Stick Popsicle through the wholes.
4. Place in the freezer for 6 hour at least. To release the Popsicle you will need to hot water from the outside of the Popsicle stick for 3 seconds. Enjoy!
Nutrition (per serving): 29 calories, | protein 0g, | carbohydrate 3g, | fiber 0g, sugar 0g, | fat 0g, | sodium 0mg | Potassium: 0mg |

Grapefruit Brûlée Breakfast Bowl

This grapefruit Brulee breakfast bowl is easy and quick to prepare.
Total time: 15minutes
Prep time: 5 minutes
Cook time: 1 0 minutes
Servings: 1
Ingredients:
1 grapefruit (peel and cut into 1/2 inch slices and cut off the bitter pith around edge of each slices)
Brown sugar
1/2 cup plain Greek yogurt
1/2 cup granola
Honey to taste
Instructions:
1. Set the oven on broiler and place a foil on a baking sheet.
2. Assemble grapefruit slices in a prepared baking sheet and dab the top of each piece with a piece of paper towel to dry up the foil.
3. Sprinkle each piece with a little brown sugar and then broil until sugar begins to bubbling, for about 10 minutes.
4. Meanwhile as the grapefruit are broiling, Combine yogurt and granola in a medium bowl and mix.
5. Add the broiled grapefruit to the yogurt mixture bowl and drizzle with honey and serve right away. Enjoy!
Nutrition (per serving): 140 calories, | protein 15g, | carbohydrate 29g, | fiber 0g, sugar 0g, | fat 4g, | sodium 0mg | Potassium: 0mg |

Spinach Feta Breakfast Wraps

Total time: 20 minutes
Prep time: 10 minutes
Cook time: 10 minutes
Servings: 4
Ingredients:
5 cup baby spinach
1/2 pint cherry or grape tomatoes, halved

10 large eggs
4 whole-wheat tortillas
4 oz. feta cheese, crumbled
2 tbsp. extra virgin olive oil
Salt to taste
Freshly ground black Pepper to taste
Instructions:
1. Crack the eggs in a large bowl and whisk until well mixed.
2. Heat oil in a large skillet over medium heat, add the eggs and cook for 2 minutes or until eggs are cooked, and stir, but not often.
3. Season with salt and pepper to taste, remove from heat and let cool to room temperature.
4. Properly rinse the skillet and place it back to the heat, add 1 tbsp. of oil and let it heat and then add the spinach, cook and stir often for about 5 minutes or until wilted
5. Remove the spinach to another plate to cool to room temperature.
6. Assemble the tortilla on a work surface and add a quarter of the eggs, tomatoes, spinach, and feta down the center of the tortilla and then wrap tightly. Repeat the process with remaining.
7. Place the wraps in a large top bag and place in the freezer until ready to serve.
 8. Wrap the burritos in aluminum foil, if you are not using within a week to avoid freezer burn.
9. Microwave on high for 2 minutes before serving.
Nutrition (per serving): 543 calories, | protein 28g, | carbohydrate 46.5g, | fiber 4.4g, sugar 3,0g, | fat 24.6g, | sodium 829.3mg | Potassium: 0mg |

Chocolate Shake Smoothie

This smoothie taste like chocolate shake smoothie, you will love it.
Total time: 5 minute
Prep time: 5 minutes
Cook time: 0 minutes
Servings: 1
Ingredients:
1 banana
1/4 avocado - peeled, pitted, and chopped
1 tbsp. flax meal
1 1/2 tbsp. cocoa powder
1/2 cup kale, ribs removed
1 cup almond milk
4 ice cubes
Instructions:

1. Combine all the ingredients in a bowl of a blender and blend until smooth.
2. Transfer smoothie in a serving glass cup serve immediately.
Nutrition (per serving): 306 calories, | protein 10g, | carbohydrate 52g, | fiber 9g, sugar 32g, | fat 2g, | sodium 229mg | Potassium: 0mg |

Citrus Green Smoothie

This recipe is loaded with vitamins and minerals and perfect for your breakfast.
Total time: 5minutes
Prep time: 5 minutes
Cook time: 0 minutes
Servings: 2
Ingredients:
1 1/2 cups almond milk
2 cups spinach frozen
2 tbsp. plant-based vanilla protein powder
1/2 large grapefruit peeled
1 cup strawberries frozen
1 orange peeled
1 banana frozen
Instructions:
1. Combine all the ingredients in a bowl of high powered blender or food processor and process until combined and smooth.
2. Divide equally among 2 serving glass cup and serve immediately.
Nutrition (per serving): 15.7calories, | protein 14g, | carbohydrate 48g, | fiber 10g, sugar 258g, | fat 4.3g, | sodium 201mg | Potassium: 839mg |

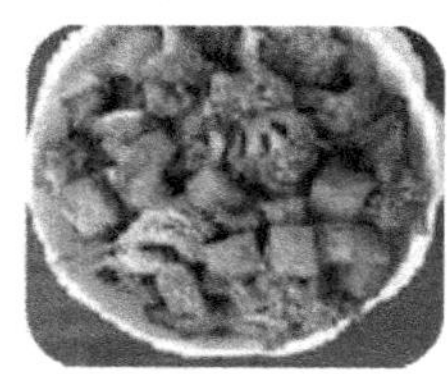

Chatpati Broccoli

Total time: 30 minutes
Prep time: 10 minutes
Cook time: 20 minutes
Servings: 2
Ingredients:
250 gm. broccoli-cut small
2 tsp. mustard seeds
2 Tbsp. extra virgin olive oil

4curry leaves
3whole red pepper
1/8 tsp. asafoetida powder
1 tsp. cumin
50 gm. ginger-shredded fine
2 tsp. garlic-chopped fine
20 gm. tamarind-soaked in 1 cup water and strained
Sea salt to taste
Instructions:
1. In skillet over medium-high heat, heat oil and add mustard, red pepper, asafetida, cumin and curry leaves, Heat oil and add mustard, curry leaves, red pepper, asafoetida and cumin and cook for 8 minutes
2. Add Ginger and garlic and cook for 3 minutes or until light brown
3. Add the broccoli and cook over high heat for 5 minutes, reduce the heat to low heat, cover and let it simmer for more 14 minutes
4. Add tamarind and season with salt and let it boil.
5. Remove from heat and serve immediately
Nutrition (per serving): 148 calories, | protein 9g, | carbohydrate 7g, | fiber 1g, sugar 3g, | fat 10g, | sodium 178mg | Potassium: 0mg |

Coffee Smoothie

This easy to make smoothie is a perfect option to start your day.
Total time: 5 minutes
Prep time: 5 minutes
Cook time: 0 minutes
Servings: 2
Ingredients:
1 cup strong brewed coffee
1/4- cup rolled oats
1 banana
1 tbsp. cocoa powder
1 tsp. honey
1 tbsp. flaxseeds meal
1/8 tsp. ground cinnamon
1 cup almond milk
Instructions:
1. Pour the coffee in an ice cube tray and freeze overnight.
2. Place the coffee ice cubes in a blender and the rest of the ingredients and blend until very smooth.
3. Taste and adjust the taste according if needed. Serve and enjoy!
Nutrition (per serving): 144 calories, | protein 3g, | carbohydrate 26g, | fiber 4g, sugar 0g, | fat 4g, | sodium 0mg | Potassium: 0mg |

Delicious Kale Smoothie

The kale smoothie is detoxifying, loaded with protein, yummy, easy and quick to prepare
Total time: 5 minute
Prep time: 2 minutes
Cook time: 3 minutes
Servings: 2
Breakfast
Ingredients:
1 banana, peel and sliced
1 cup kale
1 tbsp. unsweetened peanut butter
1 tbsp lemon juice
1 cup unsweetened almond milk
1 tbsp maple syrup
2 ice cubes
a pinch of sea salt
Instructions:
1. Combine all the ingredients in a bowl of a blender and blend until smooth and creamy.
2. Divide among 2 serving glass cup and serve immediately.
Nutrition (per serving): 203 calories, | protein 8g, | carbohydrate 33g, | fiber 0g, sugar 0g, |fat 1g, | sodium 237mg | Potassium: 0mg |

Orange Green Smoothie

This smoothies is packed with fruit and veggies
Total time: 5 minute
Prep time: 5 minutes
Cook time: 0 minutes
Servings: 1
Ingredients:
1 large orange peeled and segmented
1 frozen banana
1/2 cup unsweetened almond milk
2 cups spinach
6 frozen strawberries
1/4 cup plain Greek yogurt
Instructions:
1. Combine all the ingredients in a bowl of blender and blend until smooth and creamy
2. Transfer to a serving class cup and enjoy immediately.

Nutrition (per serving): 250 calories, | protein 10g, |carbohydrate 52g, | fiber 9g, sugar 32g, |fat 2g, | sodium 229mg |Potassium: 0mg |

Vanilla Latte Smoothie

This vanilla latte smoothie is packed with protein and flavors. You will love it.
Total time: 10 minutes
Prep time: 10 minutes
Cook time: 0 minutes
Servings: 1
Ingredients:
1 cup sugar-free vanilla almond milk
1/2 frozen banana
1 tbsp. vanilla protein powder
1 tsp. espresso powder
1/2 cup crushed ice
1/4 cup coffee flavored yogurt
1/4 tsp. pure vanilla extract
1/2 tsp. honey
Instructions:
1. Combine all the ingredients in blender and blend until smooth and creamy.
2. Transfer to a glass cup and serve immediately. Enjoy!
Nutrition (per serving): 226 calories, | protein 17g, |carbohydrate 22g, | fiber 3g, sugar0, |fat 13g, | sodium 0mg |Potassium: 0mg |

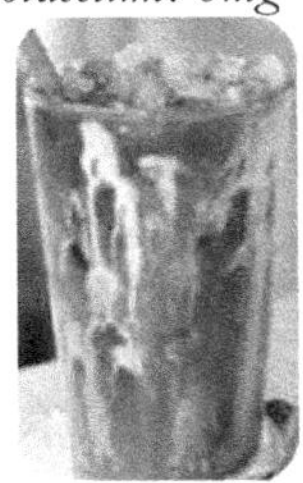

Cold Brew Mocha

This recipe is so creamy and delicious. It's perfect for starting your day.
Total time: 5 minutes
Prep time: 5 minutes
Cook time: 0 minutes
Servings: 1
Ingredients:
2/3 cup cold brew coffee
2/3 cup vanilla sugar-free almond breeze almond milk
2 cups ice cubes

1tbsp chocolate protein powder
1 tsp. cacao powder
2 medjool dates
Instructions:
1. Combine all the ingredients in a high power blender and blend until smooth and creamy.
2. Transfer to a glass cup and serve.
Nutrition (per serving): 237 calories, | protein 12g, | carbohydrate 41g, | fiber7, sugar 0g, | fat 4g, | sodium 0mg | Potassium: 0mg |

Breakfast Coffee Smoothie

This recipe is packed with whole grains, fruits and coffee.
Total time: 5 minutes
Prep time: 5 minutes
Cook time: 0 minutes
Servings: 1
Ingredients:
1 banana sliced and frozen
1/4 cup rolled oats
1/2 cup strong brewed coffee, chilled
1/2 cup almond milk
1 tsp. nut butter, optional:
Instructions:
1. Combine all the ingredients in a blender and blend until smooth and creamy
2. Transfer to a serving glass cup and enjoy.
Nutrition (per serving): 245 calories, | protein 8.1g, | carbohydrate 46.8g, | fiber 5.1g, sugar 18g, | fat 4.2g, | sodium 0mg | Potassium: 0mg |

Quick Coffee Smoothie

This coffee recipe is so easy and quick to make and it's a perfect way to your day.
Total time: 5 minutes
Prep time: 5 minutes
Cook time: 0 minutes
Servings: 1
Ingredients:
3/4 cup coffee, cooled

1/2 cup Greek yogurt

1 frozen banana

1 1/2 tbsp. vanilla protein powder

1/2 cup ice

1 tbsp. agave syrup

Instructions:

1. Combine all the ingredients in a high power blender and blend until very smooth. If you want the smoothie thicker, add more ice to get your desired consistency.

2. Transfer to glass cup and serve. Enjoy!

Nutrition (per serving): 305 calories, | protein 30g, | carbohydrate 46g, | fiber 4g, sugar 0g, |fat 0g, | sodium 0mg | Potassium: 0mg |

Avocado and Pumpkin Smoothie

This recipe is packed with protein

Total time: 10 minutes

Prep time: 5 minutes

Cook time: 0 minutes

Servings: 2

Ingredients:

2 Tbsp. ground flaxseed

1/4 avocado

7 oz. 2% Greek yogurt

1/2 cup canned pure pumpkin

1/2 cup water

1/2 tsp. pumpkin pie spice

1/2 tsp. pumpkin pie spice

Instructions:

1. Combine all the recipes in a bowl of a blender and blend until smooth and creamy.

2. Divide the smoothie among 2 serving glass cup.

Nutrition (per serving): 361 calories, | protein 26g, | carbohydrate 38g, | fiber 11g, sugar 26g, |fat 0g, | sodium 0mg | Potassium: 0mg |

Healthy Strawberry-Kiwi Smoothie

This recipe is low in calorie; using organic kiwis will make it healthier.

Total time: 10 minutes

Prep time: 5 minutes

Cook time: 0 minutes

Servings: 2

Ingredients:

1 kiwi

1 ripe banana, peel and slice
1 1/4 cup cold apple juice
5 frozen strawberries
1 1/2 teaspoon honey
Instructions:
1. Combine all the ingredients in a bowl of a blender and blend until smooth and creamy.
2. Transfer to a serving glass cup and enjoy.
Nutrition (per serving): 87 calories, | protein 0.5g, | carbohydrate 22g, | fiber 1.5g, sugar 16.5g, | fat 0g, | sodium 0mg | Potassium: 0mg |

Chocolate Frappe

This chocolate frappe is as tasty as the store bought expensive coffee, with good and less expensive ingredients.
Total time: 10 minutes
Prep time: 10 minutes
Cook time: 0 minutes
Servings: 1
Ingredients:
2 cups Ice
1 cup Cream
1/4 cup brown Sugar
1/4 cup Ghirardelli's Chocolate Syrup
For topping
Chocolate syrup and Whipped cream
Chocolate chips, optional
Instructions:
1. Combine all the ingredients in a high power blender and blend until very smooth.
2. Transfer to a serving glass cup and top with whipped cream, chocolate syrup and chocolate chips if you want. Serve immediately.
Nutrition (per serving): 142 calories, | protein 10g, | carbohydrate 41g, | fiber 5g, sugar 0g, | fat 10g, | sodium 0mg | Potassium: 0mg |

Mediterranean Breakfast Pitas

Total time: 17 minute
Prep time: 10 minutes
Cook time: 7 minutes
Servings: 4
Ingredients:
4 large eggs, at room temperature
2 whole-wheat pita breads with pockets, cut in half

1/2 cup hummus
1 medium cucumber, thinly sliced into rounds
2 medium tomatoes, large dice
Hot sauce
Handful of fresh parsley leaves, roughly chopped
Freshly ground black pepper
Sea Salt to taste

Instructions:

1. Pour water in a medium saucepan and let it boil over medium heat, add the eggs gently to the pan and cook for 7 minutes

2. Pour cold water and transfer the cooked eggs to the cold water bowl with a slotted spoon. Peel the eggs under running water and cut into 1/4 inch slices and then sprinkle with and put aside.

3. Spread each inside of the 2 pita pocket with 2 tbsp. of hummus and place tomatoes and cucumber in a each of the pita.

4. Tuck a sliced of egg into each pita sprinkle with hot sauce, parsley, salt and pepper and enjoy.

Nutrition (per serving): 206 calories, | protein 12.0g, | carbohydrate 22g, | fiber 4.9g, sugar 3.4g, | fat 8.3g, | sodium 564.4mg | Potassium: 0mg |

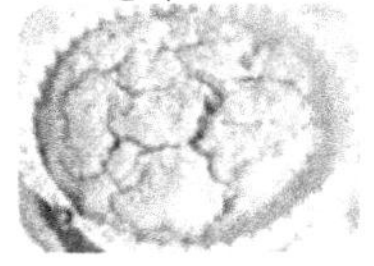

Carrot Cake Quinoa
This carrot cake is so yummy! It taste like dessert, you will love it.
Total time: 25 minutes
Prep time: 10 minutes
Cook time: 15 minutes
Servings: 16

Ingredients:
1 flax egg 1 Tbsp. flaxseed meal + 3 tbsp. water
1/4 cup pure maple syrup
1/2 cup cashew butter or nut/seed butter of choice
1 tsp. vanilla extract
1/2 cup quinoa flakes
1 medium banana mashed
1/2 cup rolled oats
1 tsp. baking powder
1/2 tsp. nutmeg
3/4 cup shredded carrots
1 tsp. cinnamon
1/4 tsp. salt

Instructions:

1. Preheat the oven to 350°F and prepare some baking sheets with parchment paper. Set aside.
2. Place the flaxseed meal in a small bowl, add water and whisk well. Set aside.
3. Combine the banana cashew butter, vanilla and syrup in a large bowl, add the flaxseed meal mixture and mix well.
4. Add the quinoa flakes, baking powder, oats, spices and salt and stir well. Add shredded carrots.
5. Place 2 tbsp. of the dough into the prepared baking sheets, continue with the dough until no more dough.
6. Place the baking sheets in the heated oven and bake until golden brown for 17 minutes.
7. Remove from oven and let it cool on the pan for 5 minutes before placing on a wire rack to cool down completely.
8. Serve warm and enjoy!

Note: Store in an air tight container and reheat slightly in the microwave before serving
Nutrition (per serving): 108 calories, | protein 2g, | carbohydrate 12g, | fiber 1g, sugar 0g, | fat 5g, | sodium 0 mg | Potassium: 0mg |

Low carb Bacon Avocado Fries

This low carb bacon avocado fries is extraordinary, you will surely love it.
Total time: 20 minutes
Prep time: 5 minutes
Cook time: 15 minutes
Servings: 24

Ingredients:

3 avocados, halved and pitted, slice each into 8 equal wedges
24 thin strips of bacon,
1/4 up ranch dressing, for serving

Instructions:

1. Preheat the oven to 425°F.
2. Wrap each avocado wedge in bacon, cut bacon if you want.
3. Place on a baking sheet, let the seam side down.
4. Bake for about 15 minutes or until bacon is crispy.
5. Remove from heat and serve with ranch dressing.

Nutrition (per serving): 120 calories, | protein 4g, | carbohydrate 3g, | fiber 2g, sugar 0g, | fat 2g, | sodium 190mg | Potassium: 0mg |

Broiled Parmesan Avocado

This recipe is loaded with nutrients and it quick to put together.

Total time: 14 minutes
Prep time: 10 minutes
Cook time: 4 minutes
Servings: 4
Ingredients:
1 avocado, halved and pitted
2 tbsp. parmesan cheese grated
1 lime juice and zest
Salt and pepper to taste
Instructions:
1. Heat toaster oven to broil.
2. Squeeze lime, Sprinkle parmesan cheese, lime zest, salt and pepper to taste over avocado
3. Broil until cheese is melted, for about 4 minutes.
4. Remove from heat and serve immediately.
Nutrition (per serving): 61 calories, | protein 4g, | carbohydrate 4g, | fiber 2g, sugar 1g, | fat 2g, | sodium 162mg | Potassium: 0mg

Bake Broccoli

This broccoli bake is so creamy and yummy!
Total time: 65 minutes
Prep time: 15 minutes
Cook time: 50 minutes
Servings: 4
Ingredients:
5 cups chopped broccoli (stems removed and cut in florets)
250 gm. cheddar cheese
1/2 pint milk
A pinch of nutmeg
3 Tbsp. plain flour
2 slices stale white bread
2-3 cloves garlic, finely chopped
1 green chili, finely chopped
1 Tbsp. extra virgin olive oil
Salt and freshly ground Black pepper taste
Instructions:
1. Preheat the oven to 400°F

2. In a pot with water, add broccoli florets and salt, cook until tender, for about 10 minutes
3. Pour the milk in a skillet and bring to a boil over medium heat.
4. Lower the heat and let it simmer, as you slowly add the flour and three quarter of the cheese
5. Add the nutmeg and garlic to the skillet and let it continue to simmer for 5 minutes
6. In a casserole dish, place the cooked broccoli and pour over the sauce.
7. Tear the bread into thumb size pieces and place over the broccoli alongside with the remaining cheese, add green chili and then season with salt and pepper to taste.
8. Add a little oil on top to make the bread crispy.
9. Place in the oven and bake until the top turns golden brown, for about 35 minutes.
10 Remove from the oven and serve warm. Enjoy!
Nutrition (per serving): 174 calories, | protein 11g, | carbohydrate 15g, | fiber 1g, sugar 2g, | fat 10g, | sodium 154mg | Potassium: 0mg |

LUNCH RECIPES

Green detox salad with Lemon Tahini Dressing

Total time: 60minutes
Prep time: 30 minutes
Cook time: 30 minutes
Servings: 4
Ingredients:
2 tbsp. tahini sesame seed paste
1 tsp. low sodium soy sauce
2 tbsp. extra virgin olive oil
1 lemon juice and zest (use 1/2 of the lemon zest)
2 tsp. fresh ginger grated
2 cloves garlic grated
Sea salt to taste
Freshly ground pepper to taste
For SALAD
1 cup unsweetened flaked coconut
2 cups cooked chickpeas
2 tbsp. low sodium soy sauce
2 tbsp. extra virgin oil
1/4 tsp. cayenne pepper
4 cups kale roughly torn

1/4 head purple cabbage shredded
2 cups fresh broccoli florets
1/2 cup fresh parsley and cilantro roughly chopped
2 red grapefruits segmented
2 ripe but firm avocados, chopped
Chia seeds and Hemp seeds for topping
For VEGAN PARMESAN
1/2 cup raw pine nuts
1 tbsp. nutritional yeast
2tsp. raw sesame seeds
Sea salt to taste
Instructions:
1. To make the lemon tahini dressing, Combine all the ingredients for the dressing in medium bowl and whisk until well mixed. You can as well make use of the food processor or blender to blend until smooth.
2. Taste and adjust salt and add pepper as needed.
3. Transfer to an air tight container with a lid and store in the fridge make sure you use within a week.
4. To make the salad, preheat the oven to 425°F
5. Spread the cooked chickpeas on a paper towel and let it completely dry for some time.
6. Add the coconut flakes and cooked dry chickpeas to a baking dish and toss with oil, soy sauce and cayenne pepper until well coat.
7. Place in the oven and roast for 20 minutes, stir and roast for more until chickpeas are brown and the coconut flake is dark brown, for about 10 minutes more.
8. Remove from heat and save any leftovers for later use.
9. In a large mixing bowl, add the kale alongside with 1 tsp. of extra virgin oil and salt to taste and then message the kale with your hands until well coated and lightly softened, for about 3 minutes.
10. Add the cabbage, broccoli, cilantro and parsley to the kale bowl and toss well. Add the dressing and toss well coated.
11. Add the chopped avocados and grapefruit segment and toss gently to combine.
12. Place the salad in the fridge for overnight or the whole day if you want.
13. In blender or food processor, combine the sesame seeds, pine nuts, nutritional yeast and a pinch of sea salt and process until crumbs that looks like parmesan cheese Is achieved. You can make this vegan parmesan ahead and store in the fridge until needed.
14. Divide the salad among 4 separate bowls and top with crunchy chickpeas and vegan parmesan cheese and then garnish with hemp seed and chia. Enjoy!

Nutrition (per serving): 232 calories, | protein 12.3g, | carbohydrate 18g, | fiber 2g, sugar19 .2g, |fat 10g, | sodium 110mg | Potassium: 0mg |

Mixed Veggies and Grapefruit Salad with Dijon Grapefruit Vinaigrette

This recipe is packed with nutrients and it's yummy!

Total time: 20 minutes
Prep time: 20 minutes
Cook time: 0 minutes
Servings: 5

Ingredients:

8 cups chopped kale (no stems)
1/2 grapefruit, peeled and segmented
1 avocado, chopped
2 Tbsp. sliced almonds

Dijon Grapefruit Vinaigrette

1 tsp. finely chopped shallot
2 Tbsp. extra-virgin olive oil
3 Tbsp. fresh grapefruit juice
2 Tbsp. extra-virgin olive oil
1/2 tsp. Dijon mustard
Sea salt to taste
Freshly ground pepper, to taste

Instructions:

1. To make the Dijon grapefruit vinaigrette, in a food processor bowl, grapefruit juice, Dijon mustard oil, shallot, salt and pepper to taste, process until smooth.

2. In a large mixing bowl, place the kale together with the vinaigrette and massage well with your hands. Transfer to a plate and let it slightly softened for about 10 minutes.

3. Arrange the grapefruit segment and chopped avocado over the kale and sprinkle with pumpkin seeds and parmesan cheese. Serve right away.

Nutrition (per serving): 71 calories, | protein 2.3g, | carbohydrate 4.2g, | fiber 0g, sugar 0.8g, |fat5.7g, | sodium 42.3mg | Potassium: 0mg |

Quick Hummus and Greek Salad

This salad recipe is quick and easy to prepare. It's loaded with nutrients.
Total time: 10 minutes
Prep time: 10 minutes
Cook time: 0 minutes
Servings: 1
Ingredients:
1/3 cup cherry tomatoes, halved
1/3 cup sliced cucumber
2 cups arugula
1 tbsp. chopped red onion
1 1/2 tbsp. extra-virgin olive oil
2 tsp. red-wine vinegar
1/8 tsp. freshly ground black pepper
1 tbsp. feta cheese
1 4-inch whole-wheat pita
1/4 cup hummus
Instructions:
1. Combine the cucumber, onion, vinegar, tomatoes oil and pepper in a serving plate and toss.
2. Top mixture with feta and serve with hummus and pita. Enjoy!
Nutrition (per serving): 422 calories, | protein 10.9g, | carbohydrate 4.9g, | fiber 7.3g, sugar 4.3g, | fat 29.9g, | sodium 485.8mg | Potassium: 543.8mg |

Lentil and Kale Salad

To make this salad recipe quicker, prepare the lentil ahead of time and refrigerate. It's takes only 15 minutes to put together.
Total time: 40 minutes
Prep time: 15 minutes
Cook time: 25 minutes
Servings: 4
Ingredients:
1/4 cup red wine vinegar
1 9-oz. package refrigerated steamed lentils
2 tbsp. extra virgin olive oil
1 tbsp. finely chopped dried tomatoes (not oil-packed)
1 clove garlic, minced
1/2 tsp. Dijon-style mustard
1/4tsp. fresh ground black pepper
1/4 cup shredded Parmesan cheese
8 cup fresh baby kale
1 cup chopped red sweet pepper

1/4 tsp. sea salt
Instructions:
1. Rinse the lentil and drain, pour 2 cups of water in a medium saucepan and let it boil over medium-high heat, add the lentil and let it boil
2. Reduce heat to low heat, cover and let it simmer until tender, for about 25 minutes. Remove from heat and let it cool.
3. Combine the oil, mustard, garlic, vinegar, dried tomatoes, salt and pepper in a large mixing bowl and whisk well.
4. Add the kale and toss to coat. Top with lentils and sweet pepper and sprinkle with cheese. Serve and enjoy.
Note: you can store the lentil in the fridge for up to 3 days

Quick Pesto Chicken Salad with Greens

You can make this recipe into a sandwich for a healthy lunch, It's loaded with nutrient and very yummy.
Total time: 30 minutes
Prep time: 10 minutes
Cook time: 20 minutes
Servings: 4
Ingredients:
1 pound boneless, skinless chicken breast, trimmed
1/4 cup pesto
1/4 cup low-fat mayonnaise
3 tbsp. finely chopped red onion
2 tbsp. red-wine vinegar
8 cup mixed salad greens
2 tbsp. Extra-virgin olive oil
1 pint grape or cherry tomatoes, halved
1/4 tsp. sea salt
1/4 tsp. ground pepper
Instructions:
1. In a saucepan over medium heat, place the chicken, pour in water, and let the water cover the chicken by 1 inch.
2. Cover the saucepan and let it boil over medium-high heat.
3. Reduce the heat to low heat and let it simmer for 15 minutes, or until chicken is no longer pink in the center.
4. Transfer chicken to a chopping board to cool and shred into small-small pieces.
5. In a medium mixing bowl. Combine the pesto, onion and mayonnaise. Add shreds chicken and toss until coated.
6. In a large mixing bowl, combine the vinegar, oil, salt and pepper and whisk well. Add the tomatoes and greens and toss to coat.

7. Divide the salad equally among 4 serving plate and top chicken salad.
Enjoy!

Nutrition (per serving): 324 calories, | protein 27.1g, |carbohydrate 9.2g, | fiber 2.3g, sugar 3.2g, |fat 19.7g, | sodium 453.9mg |Potassium: 542.2mg |

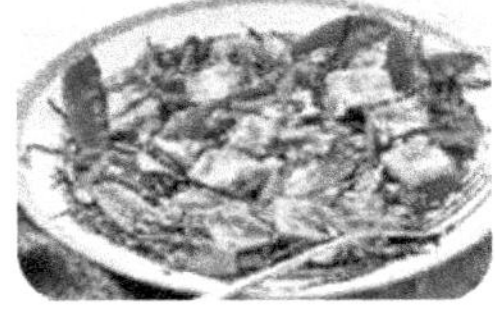

Crispy Tofu with vegetable Salad

This tofu and vegetable salad I delicious and packed with nutrients, it takes only 45 minutes to put together.

Total time: 3 hours 45 minutes
Prep time: 10 minutes
Cook time: 20 minutes
Servings: 4

Ingredients:

16-oz. package extra-firm water-packed tofu, Cut tofu crosswise into 8 equal pieces and press for 3 hours
5 tbsp. extra-virgin olive oil, divided
2 tbsp. chopped fresh basil
2 tsp. chopped fresh oregano
1/4 cup lemon juice
2 large eggs
1/4 cup all-purpose flour
2/3 cup grated Parmesan cheese
1/3 cup whole-wheat panko breadcrumbs
1/8 tsp. sea salt
1 tsp. freshly ground black pepper

For Salad

4 ripe medium sized tomatoes cut each one of them into 6 wedges
2 cups thinly sliced sweet onion
1/2 cup Castelvetrano olives
1/4 cup chopped pitted Kalamata olives
2 tbsp. Chopped fresh oregano, divided
3 tbsp. Extra-virgin olive oil
3 tbsp. chopped fresh basil, divided
2 tbsp. Red-wine vinegar
1 tbsp. Lemon juice
1/4 tsp. freshly ground black pepper
1/8 tsp.sea salt

Instructions:
1. Combine 2 tbsp. of oil, 2 tsp. of oregano, 1/4 cup of lemon juice, 2 tbsp. of tbsp. of basil, 1 tsp. of pepper and 1/8 tsp. of salt in a baking sheet.
2. Add the pressed tofu and mix until well coated, cover and put in the fridge for 2 hours or more, turn often.
3. Combine the olives, tomatoes, onion, oil, 2 tbsp. basil, 1 tsp. oregano, lemon juice, vinegar, pepper and salt in a large mixing bowl and toss well. Put salad aside, tossing occasionally.
4. Remove the tofu from the marinade, pat dry and discard the marinade. Place flour in a shallow bowl.
5. Crack the eggs in a shallow bowl and lightly beat. Combine the panko and parmesan in another shallow bowl.
6. Dip the tofu in the flour bowl, shake off any excess, dip in the egg bowl and shake off any excess and then in the panko and parmesan mixture and press well to coat.
7. In a nonstick skillet over medium heat, heat 2 tbsp. of oil until shimmering and add 1/2 of the tofu.
8. Lower the heat to low heat and cook for 4 minutes on each side or until browned, turning once.
9. Transfer to a plate lined with paper towel and then repeat the process with the remaining 1 tbsp. oil and tofu.
10. Divide the salad among 4 serving bowl and top with tofu and remaining 1 tsp. of oregano and tbsp. of basil. Enjoy!
Nutrition (per serving): 549 calories, | protein 17.6g, | carbohydrate 23g, | fiber 5.1g, sugar 6.8g, | fat 43.8g, | sodium 641.4mg | Potassium: 586.8mg |

Healthy spinach salad

With a boiled potatoes or pita chips you can turn healthy salad into a hearty vegetarian dinner. You will love it.
Total time: 1 hour 20 minutes
Prep time: 20 minutes
Cook time: 60 minutes
Servings: 8
Ingredients:
1 large Chioggia beet
1/4 cup finely chopped green garlic, white part mostly
1 cup whole-milk plain Greek yogurt
1/3 cup chopped fresh mint
4 tbsp. extra-virgin olive oil, divided
1 tbsp. butter, melted
2 tbsp. finely chopped scallion
1 tsp. dried oregano

1 pound mature spinach, finely sliced
1 tbsp. butter, melted
1 tsp. dried mint
1 tsp. ground Aleppo
1 tsp.sea salt
1/2 tsp. ground pepper
Instructions:
1. Place the beet in a saucepan, cover with water by 1 inch and bring to a boil over high heat, cook for about 50 minutes or until tender. Remove from heat and transfer to a chopping board and let it cool off. Peel and julienne the beet, when it is cooled
2. In a small saucepan over medium-low heat, heat 2 tbsp. of oil together with green garlic and cook for about 6 minutes or until garlic is soften but not brown.
3. Remove from heat and transfer to a large mixing bowl. Add the remaining 2 tbsp. of oil, fresh mint, yogurt, scallion, salt and pepper to the bowl and whisk well.
4. Add the beet to the bowl together with spinach, add the dressing and toss to coat.
5. Divide among 8 serving plate. Drizzle each plate with butter and sprinkle oregano, dried mint and Aleppo.
Note: you can cook the beet ahead of time and save in the fridge for up to 3 day.
Nutrition (per serving): 147 calories, | protein 4.4g, | carbohydrate 7.6g, | fiber 2.9g, sugar 3.8g, | fat 11.7g, | sodium 479mg | Potassium: 479.2mg |

Roasted Chicken and mushrooms Salad

This roasted chicken salad is so yummy, packed with flavor and easy to prepare.
Total time: 45 minutes
Prep time: 40 minutes
Cook time: 20 minutes
Servings: 4
Ingredients:
3 cloves garlic, minced
5 tbsp. extra-virgin olive oil
3 tsp. fennel seeds, crushed, divided
1/2 tsp. ground pepper, divided
10 oz. mushrooms, quartered
1 Ib. chicken tenders, halved crosswise
4 medium carrots, sliced 1/2 inch thick
1 medium onion, cut into 3/4-inch wedges
1 1/2 cups water
1 cup quinoa

3 tbsp. sherry vinegar or red-wine vinegar
8 cups torn escarole
1 tsp. sea salt, divided
Instructions:
1. Preheat the oven to 475°F.
2. In a small plate, place the garlic together with 3/4 tsp. of salt and mash with a knife. Transfer the mashed garlic to a large mixing bowl and add oil, 2 tsp. of fennel seeds and 1/4 tsp. of pepper and whisk well.
3. In a medium bowl, carrots, mushrooms, onion and drizzle 2 tbsp. of the oil mixture and toss well to coat.
4. Spread the veggies on a large rimmed baking dish and roast for about 10 minutes.
5. While the veggies are cooking, Place the quinoa in a saucepan, add water and let it boil over medium-high heat.
6. Reduce the heat to low heat and let it simmer for 10 minutes. Remove quinoa from heat, cover and let it stand for about 5 minutes.
7. Place the chicken in a medium bowl and add the oil mixture, 2 tsp. of oil, 1 tsp. of fennel seeds, 1/4 tsp. of salt and 1/4 tsp. of pepper and toss until coated.
8. Add the veggies, stir and nestle the chicken and among the veggies and continue to roast for more 10 minute or until chicken is cooked through.
9. Add vinegar in the remaining oil mixture and whisk well. Add escarole and quinoa to the mixture and toss well with dressing
10. To serve, top with the roasted veggies with chicken. Enjoy!
Nutrition (per serving): 516 calories, | protein 33.6g, | carbohydrate 43g, | fiber 9.7g, sugar 7.8g, | fat 23.6g, | sodium 711.2mg | Potassium: 1242mg |

Chickpea, Broccoli and Pomegranate Salad

This recipe is simple, quick to prepare and packed with flavor. I twill make a perfect lunch if serve with grilled pork, chicken or fish
Total time: 20 minutes
Prep time: 10 minutes
Cook time: 0 minutes
Servings: 6
Ingredients:
1/4cup finely sliced red onion
1/3 tsp. ground cumin
1Cup whole-milk plain yogurt
2 tbsp. tahini
2 tbsp. extra-virgin olive oil
1tbsp. Lemon juice
4 cups bite-size broccoli florets

1 can low-sodium chickpeas, rinsed cup pomegranate seeds
1/tsp. salt, divided
1. tsp. freshly ground black pepper
Instructions:
1. Pour water in a small bowl, add the onion and soak for 10 minutes, drain.
2. In a small dry skillet over medium heat, place the cumin and toast, stir for 2 minutes or until fragrant
3. Remove from heat and transfer to a large mixing bowl, add lemon juice, tahini, oil, yogurt, 1/2 tsp. of salt and pepper, whisk until well mixed.
4. Add chickpeas, broccoli, pomegranate seeds and onion to the bowl toss until well combined, let it stand for at least 10 minutes.
5. Season with the remaining 1/4 tsp. of salt and toss well. Enjoy!
Nutrition (per serving): 162 calories, | protein 6.2g, | carbohydrate 16.1g, | fiber 4.3g, sugar 3.6g, | fat 8.8g, | sodium 344.2mg | Potassium: 368.8mg |

Anchovy, Orange and Olive Salad

This recipe is easy to prepare, yummy and refreshing. You can serve with roasted chicken.
Total time: 60 minutes
Prep time: 30 minutes
Cook time: 0 minutes
Servings: 4
Ingredients:
1 small red onion, finely slice in round shape
16 black olives pitted and halved
4 small blood oranges
3 tbsp. extra-virgin olive oil
6 anchovy fillets
1 tbsp. fresh lemon juice
1/8 tsp. freshly ground black pepper
Instructions:
1. With a paring knife, peel the oranges and cut off the white pith and the membrane that covers the orange on the aside.
2. Place the orange in a plate and slice into rounds shape, make the round shape as thin as possible.
3. Assemble the slice orange in a serving plate, keep the juice aside. Add the onion all over the orange slices and top with olives followed by the anchovy fillets.
4. Add the lemon and orange juice over the mixture, drizzle oil and then sprinkle with black pepper
Pour the orange juice and lemon juice over the salad and drizzle with oil. Sprinkle with pepper.

5. Keep the salad for 30 minutes to stand at room temperature before serving.

Nutrition (per serving): 202calories, 3.1g protein, 14.6g carbohydrates, 2.8g fiber, 9.8 g sugar, 15.2g fat, 465.3mg Sodium| 236.8mg Potassium

Vegetable and Chickpea salad

This salad is packet with crispy vegetable and fresh herbs. You will love it!
Total time: 40 minutes
Prep time: 20 minutes
Cook time: 20 minutes
Servings: 6
Ingredients:
1 large eggplant, thinly sliced (slice into1/4 inch in thickness)
Salt
Extra virgin olive oil
3 Roma tomatoes, diced
1 cup cooked or canned chickpeas, drained
3 tbsp. Za'atar spice, divided
1/2 English cucumber, diced
1 cup chopped dill
1 small red onion, sliced into round shape
1 cup chopped parsley
For the Garlic Vinaigrette:
1 large lime, juice of
1-2 garlic cloves, minced
1/3 cup extra virgin olive oil
Sea Salt to taste
Freshly ground black Pepper to taste
Instructions:
1. Place the eggplant on a try and sprinkle with salt as needed. Set aside and let sit for 30 minutes.
2. Line a baking sheet with a paper bag topped with a paper towel and place closer to a stove. Pat dries the eggplant
3. Heat 5 tbsp. of oil in a skillet over medium high heat until heated, add the eggplant and cook 5 minutes turn and cook another 5 minutes or golden brown turn.
4. Remove from heat with slotted spatula and repeat the process until no more eggplant, don't over crowd the eggplant in the pan.
5. Arrange the eggplant on a try lined with paper towel to drain.
6. When you are done frying, arrange the cooled eggplant on a serving plate and sprinkle with 1 tbsp. of Za'atar.

7. In a medium bowl, combine the cucumbers, tomatoes, red onions, chickpeas, dill and parsley; add the remaining 2 tbsp. of Za'atar, and mix.
8. In small mixing bowl, combine the garlic, lime juice, oil, salt and pepper to taste and whisk well.
9. Drizzle the fried eggplant with 2 tbsp. of the dressing and then pour the rest of the dressing to the chickpea salad and mix well.
10. To serve, combine the eggplant and the chickpea in a serving plate and serve.
Nutrition (per serving): 308 calories, | protein 11.1g, | carbohydrate 17.3g, | fiber 9.6g, sugar 5.3g, | fat 15.3g, | sodium 435.5mg | Potassium: 0mg |

Tabouli with veggies salad

Total time: 20 minutes
Prep time: 20 minutes
Cook time: 0 minutes
Servings: 7
Ingredients:
1/2 cup extra-fine bulgur wheat, washed
1 English cucumber, very finely chopped
2 bunches parsley, remove part of the stems, washed, dried, and finely chopped
4 firm Roma tomatoes, very finely chopped
4 green onions, white and green parts, finely chopped
12-15 fresh mint leaves, remove the stems, washed, dried, and finely chopped
Sea Salt to taste
4 tbsp. lime juice
4 tbsp. Early Harvest extra virgin olive oil
Instructions:
1. Soak the bulgur in filtered water for 7 minute, drain and squeeze out all the liquid in it and set aside.
2. Combine the herbs, vegetables, and green onions in a large mixing bowl, add the bulgur and season to taste with salt and mix well.
3. Add the oil and lime and mix well. Cover the bowl and put in the fridge for about 30 minutes. Remove from fridge and divide among 7 plates and enjoy!
Nutrition (per serving): 190 calories, | protein 3.2g, | carbohydrate 25g, | fiber 3.1g, sugar 5.3g, | fat 10g, | sodium 435.5mg | Potassium: 0mg |

Healthy fattoush salad

This salad recipe quick, easy to make and packed with flavor.
Total time: 20 minutes

Prep time: 20 minutes
Cook time: 0 minutes
Servings: 6
Ingredients:
2 loaves pita bread
Extra Virgin Olive Oil
1/2 tsp. sumac, more for later
Sea Salt to taste
Freshly ground black pepper
1 heart of Romaine lettuce, chopped
1 cucumber, chopped
5 Roma tomatoes, chopped
5 green onions (both white and green parts), chopped
5 radishes, stems removed and thinly sliced
2 cups chopped fresh parsley leaves, remove the stems
1 cup chopped fresh mint leaves
For the Lime-vinaigrette
1 1/2 lime, juice of
1 tsp. ground sumac
1/3 cup Extra Virgin Olive Oil
1/4 tsp. ground cinnamon scant
1/4 tsp. ground allspice
Sea Salt to taste
Freshly ground black pepper to taste
Instructions:
1. Place the pita bread in a toaster oven and toast until crunchy but not
brown.
2. Heat 3 tbsp. of oil in a large saucepan; break the pita bread into pieced
and add to the oil. Fry the pita bread for 5 minutes, or until brown, tossing
often as you cook.
3. Add 1/2 tsp. of sumac, salt and pepper to the saucepan. Remove from
heat and transfer to a paper towel to drain.
4. Combine the cucumber, lettuce, green onions and tomatoes into a large
bowl together with the parsley and slice radish
5. Combine the lime juice, oil, lemon and spices in a small bowl and whisk
well.
6. Add the dress to the salad and toss gently, top with the pita chips and
toss again. Enjoy!
*Nutrition (per serving): 345calories, | protein 9.1g, | carbohydrate 39.8g, | fiber 0g,
sugar 11.4g, | fat 20.4g, | sodium 177.6mg | Potassium: 0mg |*

Veggies with chickpea salad

This salad recipe is packed with nutrients and flavor from fresh herbs, your whole family will love it.

Total time: 15 minutes
Prep time: 15 minutes
Cook time: 0 minutes
Servings: 7

Ingredients:

3 1/2 cups cooked chickpeas, drained and well rinsed
1/2 green bell pepper, cored and finely chopped
2 1/2 cups cherry tomatoes, slice in halves
3-5 green onions, both white and green parts, finely chopped
1/2 cup sun-dried tomatoes, one preserved in jars with olive oil is better
1/3 cup pitted Kalamata olives
1/2 cup freshly chopped mint or basil leaves
1/4 cup pitted green olives
1/2 cup freshly chopped parsley leaves

For Dressing

1/4 cup extra virgin olive oil
1 garlic clove, minced
2 tbsp. white wine vinegar
2 tbsp. lemon juice
1 tsp. ground sumac
1/2 tsp. Aleppo pepper
Sea Salt to taste
Freshly ground black pepper to taste

Instructions:

1. Combine the chickpeas, veggies, sun-dried tomatoes, olives, and fresh herbs in a large mixing bowl and mix well.
2. Combine the oil, lemon juice, vinegar, garlic, spices, salt and pepper to taste in a small mixing bowl and mix well.
3. Add the dressing to the salad and gently mix until coated. Cover salad bowl with a lid and put in the fridge for at least 30 minutes before serving.
4. Remove the salad from the fridge, give it a quick stir, taste and make the some necessary adjustment if possible. Enjoy!

Nutrition (per serving): 267 calories, | protein 12.4g, | carbohydrate 39,5g, | fiber 0g, sugar 8.1g, | fat 7.6g, | sodium 17.6mg | Potassium: 0mg |

Quick Shrimp Stuffed Avocados

This quick shrimp stuffed avocados is easy and quick to prepare.
Total time: 20 minutes
Prep time: 5 minutes
Cook time: 10 minutes
Servings: 6
Ingredients:
1 pound shrimp (peeled and deveined, tails removed)
1 tsp. paprika;
1 tbsp. avocado oil
2 tbsp. hot sauce
1/3 cup mayonnaise
1/2 lime juice
1/2 small red onion, finely chopped
3 avocados, halved and pits removed
2 green onions, finely sliced
Salt and pepper to taste
Instructions:
1. Place oil in a skillet and heat over medium high heat.
2. Add the shrimp and cook for 2 minutes or until shrimp is opaque.
3. Add paprika, salt and pepper tastes to the shrimp and then remove from heat and let it cool.
4. Combine hot sauce, mayonnaise, and lime juice in a bowl and mix well.
5. Scoop out the flesh in the avocado and reserve the skins.
6. Properly dice the avocado and add to another bowl, add the shrimp and red onion and toss until combined.
7. Add the mixed mayonnaise and stir gently until well coated and then season well with salt and pepper.
8. Place mixture back to the reserve avocado skins and garnish with green onions. Enjoy!

BLT Guacamole

Total time: 15 minutes
Prep time: 15 minutes
Cook time: 0 minutes
Servings: 6
Ingredients:
2 avocados, halved and pitted
4 slices bacon, cooked and chopped
1/2 cup Lettuce
1 cup cherry tomatoes, halved
1/4 cup green onions

2 limes juice
Salt and pepper to taste
Tortilla chips, for serving
1. Put the avocado in a bowl and mash until smooth buts somehow chunky.
2. Add the tomatoes, bacon green onions and lettuce to the mashed avocados, squeeze lime juice over the mixture and stir well. Season the salad mixture with salt and pepper to taste.
3. Serve alongside with tortilla chips.

DINNER RECIPES

Curry Cream Sauce Pan-Fried Salmon

Make this recipe in just 20 minutes. You can serve with basmati rice if you want, it taste so good.

Total time: 20minutes
Prep time: 5minutes
Cook time: 15 minutes
Servings: 2

Ingredients:
2 salmon fillets
1/2 cup heavy whipping cream
2 pinches ground ginger
1 tsp. mild curry powder
1 tsp. lemon juice
Sea salt and freshly ground black pepper to taste

Instructions:
1. In a skillet over medium heat, combine the cream, lemon juice, curry powder, and ginger and let it boil.
2. Lower the heat and add the salmon to the skillet cover and let simmer for 12 minutes or until fish flake easily with a fork. You can flip salmon about 2 times as you cook. Season as needed with sea salt and freshly ground pepper.
3. Remove from heat and serve. Enjoy!

Nutrition (per serving): 336 calories, | protein 22.2g, | carbohydrate 6.8g, | fiber 0g, sugar 0g, |fat 2.3g, | sodium 152.3mg |Potassium: 0mg |

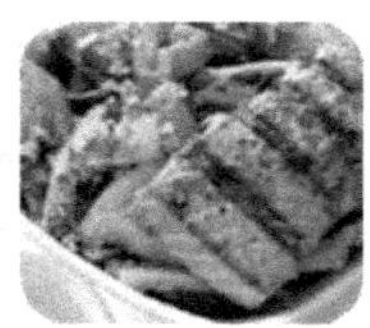

Firecracker Salmon

Marinate the salmon in the jalapeno and maple sauce and the top with more maple syrup when baking.

Total time: 55minutes
Prep time: 10 minutes
Cook time: 15 minutes
Servings: 2

Ingredients:

1/4 cup maple syrup
1 medium jalapeno (cut in half width-wise)
2 tsp. maple syrup
1 clove garlic, minced
1 tbsp. rice wine vinegar
2 fillets salmon fillets
Sea salt and freshly ground pepper to taste

Instructions:

1. Preheat the oven to 425°F and place parchment paper on a baking sheet
2. In a bowl of food processor or blender, combine 1/2 jalapeno pepper, garlic, 1/4 cup of maple syrup, vinegar, sea salt and pepper to taste and process until smooth.
3. In a large zip log bag, place the salmon fillets and pour in the mixture, seal and put in the fridge for 20 minutes.
4. Remove from fridge and let it sit at room temperature for 10 minutes.
5. Remove the salmon fish from marinade and pat dry with paper towel and Place in the baking sheet, season with sea salt and freshly ground pepper.
6. Add the rest of the jalapeno pepper on top of the salmon fish then and bake for 10 minutes
7. Remove from oven and brush the salmon fillet with 2 tsp. of maple syrup and return to the oven and bake for more 5 minutes or until fish flake easily with fork.
8. Remove from oven and serve. Enjoy!

Nutrition (per serving): 366 calories, | protein 36g, | carbohydrate 31.9g, | fiber 0g, sugar 0g, | fat 10g, | sodium 732mg | Potassium: 0mg |

Pistachio-Crusted Salmon

This recipe is quick and easy to prepare. You can make it for your dinner pretty.

Total time: 25minutes
Prep time: 10minutes
Cook time: 15 minutes
Servings: 4
Ingredients:
1 tbsp. grated Parmesan cheese
1/4 cup crushed pistachios
2 tbsp. panko bread crumbs
1 tbsp. Butter, melted
4 fillets salmon with skin, center cut
1 tbsp. Dijon mustard
Sea salt and freshly ground black pepper to taste
2 tbsp. extra virgin olive oil
4 lemon wedges
Instructions:
1. Preheat the oven to 375°F
2. In medium bowl, combine the pistachios, Parmesan cheese, panko bread crumbs, butter and whisk until well mixed.
3. Properly seasoned the salmon fillets with sea salt and freshly ground pepper on both side to taste.
4. In a large oven-save skillet, heat oil on medium-high heat. Place the salmon fillets skin side down and sear for about 3 minutes.
5. Top the salmon fillet with the pistachio mixture and press down.
6. Place the in the oven and bake for 12 minutes or until salmon flake easily.
7. Remove from oven and serve with lemon wedges
Note: Chop the pistachios in a food processor
Nutrition (per serving): 459 calories, | protein 36.2g, | carbohydrate 6.8g, | fiber 10g, sugar 25g, | fat 32g, | sodium 322.3mg | Potassium: 0mg |

Salmon Foil-Pack

This recipe can be made as a last minutes dinner idea and you can as well make it ahead of the time
Total time: 30minutes
Prep time: 10minutes
Cook time: 20 minutes
Servings: 1
Ingredients:
1 salmon fillet
2 sheets nonstick aluminum foil
1 small yellow squash, cut into 1/4-inch rounds
1 small sweet potato, peeled and sliced into 1/4-inch slices
1 small zucchini, cut into 1/4-inch rounds

1 1/2 tsp. smoky mesquite seasoning
1 lemon, cut into wedges
Instructions:
1. Preheat the oven to 400°F
2. Prepare 2 large squares of foil, the nonstick side up and let the one be on top of other.
3. Layer Zucchini, potato and squash in the center of the foil in the top and then season each layer with mesquite season.
4. Place the salmon fillet on the layer and fold over the foil and then seal the packet tightly.
5. Place in the oven and bake for 20 minutes or until salmon fillet flake easily with fork.
6. Remove from oven and Serve with lemon wedges.
Nutrition (per serving): 377 calories, | protein 35.6g, | carbohydrate 40.4g, | fiber 0g, sugar 0g, |fat 9.1g, | sodium 1522mg | Potassium: 0mg | |

Delicious Raw Bean Salad

This raw bean is quick and easy to prepare, so yummy!
Total time: 25 minutes
Prep time: 25 minutes
Cook time: 0 minutes
Servings: 4
Ingredients:
1/2 cup packed fresh basil leaves
3 tbsp. red-wine vinegar
1 tbsp. finely chopped shallot
2 tsp. Dijon mustard
1/4 cup extra-virgin olive oil
1 tsp. honey
1 cans low-sodium cannellini beans, rinsed
1/2 cucumber, halved lengthwise and sliced
10 cups mixed salad greens
1 cup halved cherry or grape tomatoes
1/4tsp. sea salt
1/4 tsp. freshly ground pepper

Instructions:
1. In a food processor or blender, combine the vinegar, basil, oil, mustard, shallot, honey, salt and pepper and process until almost smooth.
2. Transfer mixture to a large mixing bowl, add the beans, greens, cucumber and tomatoes and then toss until well coated.
3. Divide among 4 serving plate and enjoy!

Nutrition (per serving): 246 calories, | protein 7.5g, | carbohydrate 21.5g, | fiber 7.6g, sugar 4.9g, | fat 15.3g, | sodium 270.5mg | Potassium: 793.3mg |

Chicken & Farro Herb Salad

This recipe is packed with flavor, so healthy!

Total time: 60 minutes

Prep time: 20 minutes

Cook time: 40 minutes

Servings: 6

Ingredients:

1 1/2 tbsp. Dijon mustard

1 small clove garlic, minced

3/4 tsp. Kosher salt

1/2 tsp. ground pepper

1/3 cup red-wine vinegar

1/2 cup extra-virgin olive oil

For Salad

3 cups water

1 1/2 pounds boneless, skinless chicken breast, trimmed

1 cup farro

1 fennel bulb, cored and chopped

1 cup diced carrot

1 cup chopped seeded English cucumber

1/2 cup finely chopped red onion

1/4 cup chopped flat-leaf parsley

1/4 cup fresh basil, finely sliced

2 cups arugula, tough stems removed, coarsely chopped

1/4 cup oil-cured black olives, sliced

1/4 cup fresh mint, finely sliced

1/2 tsp. Sea salt

1/4 tsp. freshly ground black pepper

Instructions:

1. Combine the mustard, vinegar, garlic in a small mixing bowl and whisk well. Season the mixture with 3/4 tsp. of sea salt and 1/2 tsp. of freshly ground pepper. Add oil and whisk well.

2. In a saucepan over medium, pour in water and bring to a boil, add the farro to the pan.

3. Reduce the heat low heat, cover with a lib and let it simmer until tender, for about 25 minutes.

4. Remove from heat, drain and transfer to a large mixing bowl

5. Add 1/3 cup of vinaigrette to the farro and toss. Let it cool.

6. Preheat the grill to medium-high. Sprinkle the chicken with sea and freshly black pepper; coat the grill rack with oil.

7. Place the seasoned chicken on the grill rack and grill for 15 minutes, turn chicken once or twice or until chicken golden brown. Remove from heat and let cool before slicing.

8. Add carrot, cucumber, onion, fennel, mint, parsley, basil, and 1/3 cup of vinaigrette into the farro bowl.

9. To serve, Divide farro mixture into 6 serving plate and stir in arugula, top with sliced chicken, olives and rest of the vinaigrette. Enjoy!

Nutrition (per serving): 459 calories, | protein 28.2g, | carbohydrate 28g, | fiber 5.3g, sugar 4.8g, | fat 24.5g, | sodium 512.6mg | Potassium: 529.9mg |

Pita Bread & Hummus Mixed Green Salad

This recipe super quick to make and loaded with nutrients.

Total time: 10 minutes

Prep time: 10 minutes

Cook time: 0 minutes

Servings: 1

Ingredients:

2 cups mixed salad greens

1 1/2 tsp. extra-virgin olive oil

1/2 cup sliced cucumber

2 tbsp. grated carrot

1 1/2 tsp. balsamic vinegar

1 6 1/2-inch whole-wheat pita bread, toasted

1/4 cup hummus

Pinch of sea salt

Pinch of freshly ground black pepper

Instructions:

1. Combine the cucumber, greens and carrot in a medium plate and drizzle with vinegar and oil.

2. Sprinkle the mixture with a pinch of sea salt and black pepper.

3. Serve salad with hummus and pita.

Nutrition (per serving): 374 calories, | protein 13.5g, | carbohydrate 52.6g, | fiber 10.7g, sugar 5.3g, | fat 14.5g, | sodium 759.8mg | Potassium: 732,1mg |

Yummy cedar Planked Salmon

This recipe is packed with nutrients. You will live it.

Total time 35minutes
Prep time: 15minutes
Cook time: 20 minutes
Servings: 6
Ingredients:
2 salmon fillets, remove skin
3 untreated cedar planks (12")
1 tsp. sesame oil
1/3 cup extra virgin olive oil
1 1/2 tbsp. rice vinegar
1/3 cup soy sauce
1/4 cup chopped green onions
1 tbsp. grated fresh ginger root
1 tsp. minced garlic
Instructions:
1. Pour warm water in medium bowl and add the cedar planks and let it soak for 1 hour or more, if possible.
2. Combine the olive oil, rice vinegar, green onions, ginger, garlic sesame oil, soy sauce in a shallow dish and stir well.
3. Put the salmon fish in the mixture and turn well coat. Cover and let it marinate for 30 minutes to 1 hour.
4. Preheat the grill gas to medium heat and place the cedar planks on the grate. When the board start to smoke and crackle that shows that it is ready.
5. Remove the salmon fish from the marinade and discard the marinade. Place the salmon fish onto the cedar planks and cover.
6. Place in a grill rack and bake for 20 minutes or until fish flake easily with fork.
7. Remove from heat and serve. Enjoy!
Nutrition (per serving): 678 calories, | protein 61.3g, | carbohydrate 1.7g, | fiber 0g, sugar 0g, | fat 45.8g, | sodium 981.2mg | Potassium: 0mg |

Quick delicious Maple Salmon

This maple salmon recipe is super delicious and quick to prepare. Your whole family will love it

Total time30minutes plus more 30 minutes
Prep time: 10 minutes
Cook time: 20 minutes
Servings:4
Ingredients:
1Ib. salmon
1/4 cup maple syrup
2 tbsp. soy sauce

1 clove garlic, minced
1/4 tsp. garlic salt
1/8 tsp. freshly ground black pepper
Instructions:
1. Preheat oven 400°F
2. Combine the soy sauce, maple syrup, garlic, salt, and pepper and mix
well.
3. Put the salmon fish in a glass baking dish, add the soy sauce mixture and
mix until well coated, cover and put in the fridge for about 30 minutes.
4. Place the in the heated oven and bake for uncovered until fish flake
easily with fork, for about 20 minutes.
5. Remove from heat and serve.
*Nutrition (per serving): 265 calories, | protein 23.2g, | carbohydrate 14.1g, | fiber 0g,
sugar 0g, | fat 45.8g, | sodium 633.1mg | Potassium: 0mg |*

Bruschetta Chicken Stuffed Avocados

This recipe can be prepared in 10 minutes and it taste so good.
Total time: 10 minutes
Prep time: 10 minutes
Cook time: 0 minutes
Servings: 4
Ingredients:
3 Ripe and firm avocados (cut in halve, pits and skin removed)
1/2 Juice of 1/2 lemon
2 cup cooked and shredded chicken
1/4 red onion, finely chopped
1/4 tsp. red pepper flakes
2 large tomatoes, diced
1 tbsp. avocado oil
Kosher salt
Freshly ground black pepper
For Garnish
Thinly sliced basil
Balsamic glaze
Directions
1. Squeeze the lemon juice all over the avocado to avoid browning.
2. Combine the chicken, red onion, tomatoes, avocado oil, red pepper
flakes, salt and pepper in a large bowl and mix well.
3. Spoon the chicken mixture into the avocados and then drizzle the
balsamic glaze over the chicken mixture. Garnish with sliced basil. Serve
and enjoy

Baked Dijon Salmon

This is a perfect way to roast your salmon fish, it is so yummy. Your whole family will love it.

Total time 35minutes

Prep time: 20 minutes

Cook time: 15 minutes

Servings: 4

Ingredients:

1/4 cup butter, melted

3 tbsp. Dijon mustard

1 1/2 tbsp. honey

1/4 cup finely chopped pecans

1/4 cup dry bread crumbs

4 tsp. chopped fresh parsley

4 salmon fillets

1 lemon, for garnish

Sea salt to taste

Freshly ground pepper to taste

Instructions:

1. Preheat the oven to 400°F

2. Combine the mustard, butter, and honey in a mixing bowl and mix well. Set aside

3. In another bowl, combine the pecans, parsley and bread crumbs and mix well.

4. Brush each salmon fish with the mustard mixture and then sprinkle with the pecans mixture.

5. Place in the oven and bake until fish flake easily with for, for about 15 minutes.

6. Remove from the oven and season with salt and pepper to taste and garnish with wedge of lemon. Enjoy!

Nutrition (per serving): 422 calories, | protein 24.3g, | carbohydrate 17.6g, | fiber 0g, sugar 0g, | fat 29g, | sodium 480.3mg | Potassium: 0mg |

Pan Seared Salmon

This recipe is quick and easy to prepare and taste yummy.

Total time20 minutes

Prep time: 10 minutes

Cook time: 10 minutes

Servings: 4

Ingredients:

4 salmon fillets

2 tbsp. capers

2 tbsp. extra virgin olive oil
1/8 tsp. salt
1/8 tsp. freshly ground black pepper
Instructions:
1. Preheat a large skillet over medium-high heat for about 3 minutes.
2. Properly coat the salmon fish with oil and place in the heated skillet.
3. Increase the heat to high heat and cook for 3 minutes. Sprinkle fish with caper, salt and pepper.
4. Turn the salmon fish over and cook until fish turns brown and flake easily with fork, for about 5 minutes more.
5. Divide among 4 serving plate and garnish with lemon slices.
Nutrition (per serving): 371 calories, | protein 33.7g, | carbohydrate 1.7g, | fiber 0g, sugar 0g, | fat 25.1g, | sodium 299.8mg | Potassium: 0mg |

Blackened Salmon Fillets

This recipe is super easy and taste so good.
Total time 25 minutes
Prep time: 15 minutes
Cook time: 10 minutes
Servings: 4
Ingredients:
1 tbsp. ground cayenne pepper
1tbsp.Onion powder
1/2tsp. ground white pepper
1/4 tsp. dried oregano
2 tbsp. ground paprika
1/4 tsp. dried basil
4 salmon fillets, Remove skin and bones
1/4 tsp. dried thyme
1/2 cup unsalted butter, melted
2 tsp. Sea salt
1/2 tsp. freshly ground black pepper
Instructions:
1. Combine the paprika, onion powder, cayenne pepper, oregano thyme, basil, white pepper, salt and black pepper in a mixing bowl and mix well.
2. Properly brush the salmon fish wit 1/4 cup of butter and evenly sprinkle with the mixture. Drizzle one side of the salmon fish with rest of the butter.
3. Cook salmon fish in a skillet over medium- high heat let the butter side down, cook for 5 minutes or until browned and easily flakes with fork.
4. Remove from heat and serve.
Nutrition (per serving): 511 calories, | protein 37.4g, | carbohydrate 4.5g, | fiber 0g, sugar 0g, | fat 38.3g, | sodium 1248.4mg | Potassium: 0mg |

Balsamic-Glazed Salmon Fillets

This recipe is extraordinary yummy.
Total time30minutes
Prep time: 20minutes
Cook time: 10 minutes
Servings:6
Ingredients:
6 salmon fillets (5 oz.)
1 tbsp. white wine
1 tbsp. Honey
1/3 cup balsamic vinegar
4 tsp. Dijon mustard
1 tbsp. Chopped fresh oregano
4 cloves garlic, minced
Sea salt to taste
Freshly ground pepper to taste
Instructions:
1. Preheat the oven to 400°F and place aluminum foil on a baking dish and lightly coated with non-stick cooking spray.
2. Spray saucepan with non-stick cooking spray and place over medium heat, add garlic, stir and cook for 3 minutes or until softened.
3. Add in balsamic vinegar, white wine, honey, mustard, salt and pepper and let it simmer uncovered until slightly thickened.
4. Assemble salmon fish on prepared baking dish and properly brush with glaze, balsamic and then sprinkle with oregano
5. Place in the oven and bake until fish flake easily with fork for 10 minutes. Brush fish with rest of the glaze and season with salt and pepper.
6. Remove the fish from oven and transfer to serving plate, leave the skin on the foil. Enjoy!
Nutrition (per serving): 288 calories, | protein 28.5g, | carbohydrate 6.5g, | fiber 0g, sugar 0g, | fat 15.5g, | sodium 171.2mg | Potassium: 0mg |

Alaska Salmon Bake with Pecan Crunch Coating

This bakes salmon yummy and satisfying!
Total time 30 minutes
Prep time: 10 minutes
Cook time: 20 minutes
Servings: 6
Ingredients:
6 salmon fillets
5 tsp. honey
3 tbsp. Dijon mustard

3 tbsp. Butter, melted
1/2 cup fresh bread crumbs
1/2cup finely chopped pecans
3 tsp. chopped fresh parsley
Sea salt taste
Freshly ground pepper to taste
6 lemon wedges
Instructions:
1. Preheat the oven to 400°F and place aluminum foil on a baking dish and lightly grease with cooking oil.
2. Combine the honey mustard and butter in a small mixing bowl and mix well.
Set aside.
3. Combine the pecans, parsley, bread crumbs in another small mixing bowl
4. Properly season each salmon fillet with salt and pepper. Place the season salmon fillet on a prepared baking dish.
5. Brush with mustard mixture and cover the top of each fish with pecans mixture
6. Place in the oven and bake for 10 minutes on each side or until fish flake easily with fork.
7. Remove from the oven and garnish with lemon wedges and enjoy.
Nutrition (per serving): 368 calories, | protein 26.1g, | carbohydrate 15.9g, | fiber 0g, sugar 0g, |fat 22.4g, | sodium 352.9mg |Potassium: 0mg |

Lemon Rosemary Salmon

This lemon rosemary salmon fish is quick and easy to prepare, it is perfect for your dinner. Make for 2
Total time 30 minutes
Prep time: 10 minutes
Cook time: 20 minutes
Servings: 4
Ingredients:
2 salmon fillets, bones and skin removed
1 lemon, finely sliced
1 tbsp. extra virgin olive oil
4 sprigs fresh rosemary
Sea salt to taste
Instructions:
1. Preheat the oven to 400°F
2. In baking sheet, arrange 1/2 of the lemon slices in a single layer.

3. Layer with 2 rosemary, place lemon fish on top and sprinkle with salt,
Layer with the rest of the lemon slices and drizzle with oil.
4. Place in the oven and bake until fish flakes easily with fork, for about 20
minutes.
5. Remove from the oven and serve with crusty bread and salad.
*Nutrition (per serving): 257calories, | protein 20.5g, |carbohydrate 6.1g, | fiber 0g,
sugar 0g, |fat 18g, | sodium 1106.7mg | Potassium: 0mg |*

Chocolate Covered Grapefruit

This chocolate and grapefruit combination is so yummy and irresistible
Total time: 30minutes
Prep time: 30 minutes
Cook time: 0 minutes
Servings: 30 pieces
Ingredients:
1 Ib. melting dark chocolate
 3 red grapefruits, peeled and segmented
Instructions:
1. Place the dark chocolate in a bowl and carefully dip the segmented
grapefruit in the chocolate, dip one at a time, let the excess drip off.
2. Place the coated grapefruit on a paper towel lined baking sheets
3. Place the baking sheet in the fridge for at least 10 minutes before serving.
Enjoy!
*Nutrition (per serving): 170 calories, | protein 2.5g, |carbohydrate 20g, | fiber 1.3g,
sugar 17.4g, |fat 9g, | sodium 24mg |Potassium: 0mg |*

Salmon turmeric Soup Recipe

This salmon turmeric is well spiced with lot of fresh herbs.
Total time: 25 minutes
Prep time: 10 minutes
Cook time: 30 minutes
Servings: 4
Ingredients:
1 tsp. cumin
1/2 tsp. red pepper flakes
1 1/2 tsp. coriander
3/4tsp. turmeric
1 1/2Ib.salmon fish fillet cut into 1 1/2 -inch pieces
1/2 tsp. Paprika
Kosher salt and black pepper
Extra virgin olive oil
1 red onion, finely chopped

4 garlic cloves minced
1 red bell pepper, finely chopped
1/2 cup white wine
2 celery ribs, finely chopped
4 cups vegetable broth, preferably low-sodium
1 28- oz. can whole tomatoes
1 cup packed chopped fresh parsley
1 lemon juice
1 cup packed chopped fresh cilantro
3 green onions chopped (both white and green parts)

Instructions:

1. Combine all the spices together in a small mixing bowl and mix well.
2. Season the salmon with a pinch of salt and pepper, add 3 tsp. of mixed spices and toss until well coated.
3. Heat 3 tbsp. of oil in large pot over medium-high heat and add onions, garlic, celery, bell peppers to the pot and cook, tossing frequently until veggies is soften, about for 5 minutes.
4. Add the rest of the spices mixture and season with a pinch of salt and freshly ground black pepper.
5. Add the white wine, tomatoes, and vegetable broth to the pot and let it boil over medium-high heat.
6. Reduce the heat to low heat, cover the pot a lid partially and let it simmer for 20 minutes
7. Add the salmon and cook until fish flakes easily with a fork for about 5 minutes
8. Add the cilantro, green onions, parsley to the pot and stir well.
9. Serve with lemon juice. Enjoy!

Note: Store the leftover in the fridge for up to 2 days or more reheat before serving.
Nutrition (per serving): 207 calories, | protein 26g, | carbohydrate 16.6g, | fiber 4.2g, sugar 0g, | fat 2.1g, | sodium 0mg | Potassium: 1285.7mg |

Quinoa Cucumber Salad

This salad recipe is packed with lot of fresh vegetable and it quick and easy to put together.

Total time: 15 minutes
Prep time: 15 minutes

Cook time: 0 minutes
Servings: 6
Ingredients:
6 tbsp. red-wine vinegar
3 tbsp. chopped fresh oregano
1 1/2 tsp. Dijon mustard
1/4 tsp. crushed red pepper
3 cups cooked quinoa, cooled
1 cup crumbled feta, divided
1 cup halved grape tomatoes
2 cups thinly cucumber
1 1/2 tbsp. honey
1 1/2 cups thinly sliced red onion
1/2 cup extra-virgin olive oil
1/2 cup halved pitted Kalamata olives
1 cans no-salt-added chickpeas, rinsed
3 cups baby spinach
Instructions:
1. Combine the olive oil, oregano, vinegar, honey, Dijon and red pepper
into large mixing bowl and whisk well.
2. Add the quinoa, onion, tomatoes, cucumber, chickpeas, olives and 1/2 of
cup feta to the bowl and toss until well combined.
3. Cover bowl with a lid and put in the fridge for 30 minutes.
4. Remove from the fridge and add the spinach, toss to combine. Sprinkle
with the remaining 1/2 cup of feta and right away. Enjoy!
*Nutrition (per serving): 472 calories, | protein 12.1g, | carbohydrate 39.1g, | fiber
6.92g, sugar7.4 g, |fat 30.1g, | sodium 393.3mg | Potassium: 106.6mg |*

Broccoli, Quinoa & Chicken Salad

*This broccoli quinoa and chicken recipe is loaded with flavor and it's super healthy and
easy to make.*
Total time: 35 minutes
Prep time: 35 minutes
Cook time: 0 minutes
Servings: 4
Ingredients:
1 boneless, skinless chicken breast, trimmed
8 oz. Broccoli with stems, Trim, peel and finely slice the stem and chop the
florets into bit sizes.
2 small lemons, thinly sliced and seeded, chop 1/2 of the lemon slices.
4 tbsp. extra-virgin olive oil, divided into two
1/8 tsp. Sea salt plus 1/4 tsp. divided into two

1 cup low-sodium chicken broth
1/2 cup quinoa
3/4 cup chopped walnuts, toasted
1/4 cup red-wine vinegar
1 tbsp. Dijon mustard
2 cups arugula
1/2 cup dried cranberries
1/2 cup chopped fresh mint
Instructions:
1. Preheat the oven to 425°F. Place the chicken on one side of the baking
dish and drizzle with1 tbsp. of oil, sprinkle with 1/8 tsp. of sea salt.
2. Place the baking dish in the oven and roast for 10 minutes. On the other
side of the baking dish, place the lemon slice and roast until chicken is
cooked through and turn golden brown, for about 10 more minutes.
3. In a small saucepan over medium-high heat, place the quinoa together
with the chicken broth and let it boil.
4. Reduce heat to low, cover with a lid and let it simmer for about 15
minutes or until the liquid is absorbed. Remove from heat and let it sit for
at least 10 minutes.
4. Combine mustard, vinegar and the remaining 3 tbsp. of olive oil and 1/4
tsp. of sea salt. In a large mixing bowl
5. Shred the chicken and add to the bowl, add the broccoli, arugula
cranberries, walnuts, quinoa remaining lemon slices and mint to the
dressing bowl and toss until well combined. Enjoy!
*Nutrition (per serving): 481 calories, | protein 21.5g, | carbohydrate 43g, | fiber 7.9g,
sugar 18.8g, |fat 26.5g, | sodium 365.5mg |Potassium: 5845mg |*

Vegetable and white bean salad

*This salad is packed with flavor and satisfying, you can add any seasonal veggies of
choice.*
Total time: 10 minutes
Prep time: 10 minutes
Cook time: 0 minutes
Servings: 1
Ingredients:
3/4 cup chopped cucumbers
1/2 avocado, diced
1 tbsp. red-wine vinegar
2 cups mixed salad greens
1/3 cup canned white beans, rinsed and drained
2 tsp. extra-virgin olive oil
1/4tsp. Sea salt

Freshly ground pepper black to taste
Instructions:
1. In a mixing bowl, combine the cucumbers, greens, avocado and beans.
2. Drizzle salad with oil and vinegar and olive oil and season with sea salt and black pepper and toss until well mixed.
3. Transfer to a serving plate and enjoy.
Nutrition (per serving): 360 calories, | protein 10.1g, | carbohydrate 29.7g, | fiber 13.3g, sugar 2.9g, | fat 22.6g, | sodium 321.3mg | Potassium: 1291.6mg |

Quinoa chicken Salad

This salad is loaded with nutrition and very easy to make. It is satisfying when you make it in the evening and pack the rest for lunch.
Total time: 40 minutes
Prep time: 20 minutes
Cook time: 0 minutes
Servings: 4
Ingredients:
1/2 tsp. garlic powder
1/2 red onions, cut into 1/4-inch-thick wedges
1 medium sweet potato, peeled and cut into 1/2-inch-thick wedges
2 tbsp. Extra-virgin olive oil, divided
8 oz. chicken tenders
2 tbsp. Whole-grain mustard, divided
1 tbsp. Finely chopped shallot
1 tbsp. pure maple syrup
1 tbsp. cider vinegar
4 cups mixed baby greens, like kale, arugula and spinach, washed and dried
1/2 cup cooked and cooled red quinoa
1 tbsp. unsalted sunflower seeds, toasted
1/4 tsp. sea salt, divided
Instructions:
1. Preheat the oven to 425°F.
2. In a medium bowl, combine the sweet potato, 1tbsp. of oil, onion, garlic and 1/8 tsp. sea salt and toss well.
3. Spread mixture in a large rimmed baking sheet and roast until potato is tender, for about 15 minutes.
4. While the potato mixture is roasting, add chicken and 1 tbsp. mustard to a medium bowl and toss until coated.
5. Remove the potato mixture from the oven and stir well. Add the chicken to the baking sheet and return to the oven and roast for another 10 minutes or until chicken is cooked through and vegetable start to turn brown.
Remove from the oven and it cool off.

6. In a large mixing bowl, combine the maple syrup, shallot, the remaining 1 tbsp. of mustard, 1 tbsp. of olive oil, 1/8 tsp. of sea salt and whisk well.
7. Shred the chicken when it is cooled and add to the dressing bowl. Add quinoa, baby greens and roasted veggies to the bowl and toss well, sprinkle with the sunflower seeds and serve, enjoy!
Nutrition (per serving): 466 calories, | protein 28.7g, | carbohydrate 35.4g, | fiber 5.5g, sugar 11.6g, | fat 21.1g, | sodium 716mg | Potassium: 665.8mg |

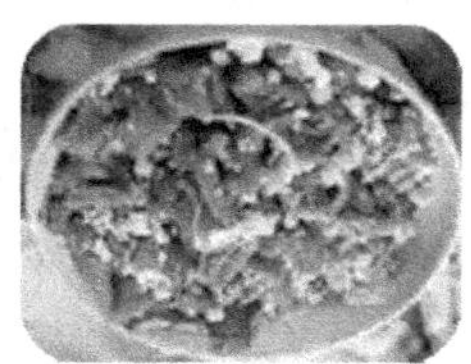

Olive, Watermelon, Feta &Caper Salad

This mixed fruit salad is sweet and savory; in just 30 minutes you are done.
Total time: 30 minutes
Prep time: 30 minutes
Cook time: 0 minutes
Servings: 6
Ingredients:
1/4 cup rinsed capers
1/3 cup pitted Kalamata olives, halved
2 tbsp. extra-virgin olive oil plus 1/4 cup, divided
1 1/2 tbsp. sherry vinegar
1/2 cup finely sliced fresh basil
2/3 cup coarsely cbled feta cheese
5 cups diced watermelon
1/2 cup finely sliced fresh mint
1/4 cup sliced almonds, lightly toasted
Flaky sea salt for garnish
Ground pepper to taste

Instructions:
1. In a small saucepan over medium-high heat, heat 2 tbsp. of oil pat dry the capers and add to the pan, cook and stir for about 3 minutes or until crisp.
2. Transfer to a plate line with a paper towel. Using a slotted spoon, and then threw away the oil
3. In a large mixing bowl, combine the vinegar, olives, watermelon, mint, basil, pepper and the remaining 1/4 cup of oil and gently toss until well coated.

4. Assemble in a large shallow serving bowl, sprinkle almonds, feta and the capers and then sprinkle a little salt and enjoy.
Nutrition (per serving): 260 calories, | protein 4.4g, | carbohydrate 12.7g, | fiber 1.8g, sugar 8.7g, | fat 22.1g, | sodium 356 mg | Potassium: 228.5mg |

Spiralized Crisp Cucumber Salad

This crisp cucumber recipe is healthy and quick to prepare.
Total time: 20 minutes
Prep time: 20 minutes
Cook time: 0 minutes
Servings: 6
Ingredients:
1 large cucumber (cut lengthwise "noodles" with spiral vegetable slicer with the chipper blade attachment) cut the noodles into 2" lengths
1/4 cup extra-virgin olive oil
1/2cup cubed feta cheese
2 tbsp. red-wine vinegar
1 cup halved cherry tomatoes
1/2 cup thinly sliced red onion
1/4 cup sliced pitted Kalamata olives
1 tbsp. Chopped fresh oregano
1/4 tsp. sea salt
1/4 tsp. freshly ground black pepper
Instructions:
1. Combine the vinegar, oil, oregano, salt and pepper in a large mixing bowl and whisk.
2. Add the olives, cucumber noodles, tomatoes, onion and cheese to vinegar mixture bowl and toss until well coated.
3. Serve Immediately
Nutrition (per serving): 149 calories, | protein 2.6g, | carbohydrate 4.9g, | fiber 0.8g, sugar 2.5g, | fat 13.4g, | sodium 291.8mg | Potassium: 169.2mg |

FISH AND SEAFOOD

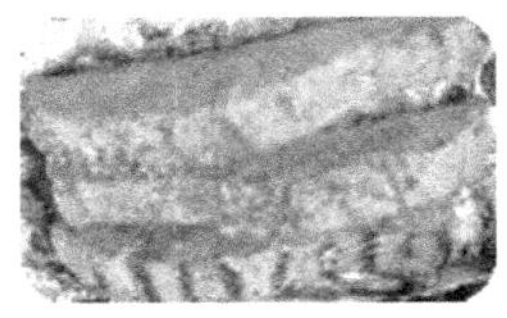

Quick Salmon with Ginger Glaze

This recipe is so quick and easy to prepare and so yummy.
Total time: 25minutes
Prep time: 5 minutes
Cook time: 20 minutes
Servings: 2
Ingredients:
4 fresh salmon fillets
1/3 cup cold water
1/4 cup seasoned rice vinegar
1 tbsp. hot Chile paste
4 cloves garlic, minced
1 tsp. soy sauce
1 tbsp. finely grated fresh ginger
2 tbsp. brown sugar
Sea salt to taste
1/4 cup chopped fresh basil
Instructions:
1. Preheat the grill to medium heat and coat the grate lightly with cooking oil.
2. Properly seasoned the salmon fillet with sea salt as needed
3. Place the seasoned salmon fillet on a preheated grill and coo cook for 15 minutes, turn the salmon fillet once at middle of the time.
4. In small saucepan, combine the rice vinegar, garlic, brown sugar, chile paste, ginger, soy sauce and water and cook over medium heat and let it boil.
5. Lower the heat and let it simmer for 5 minutes or until almost thickened.
6. Sprinkle basil on top salmon and top glaze over the basil.
Nutrition (per serving): 377calories, | protein 48.4g, | carbohydrate 13.4g, | fiber 0g, sugar 0g, | fat 13.7g, | sodium 519.1mg | Potassium: 0mg |

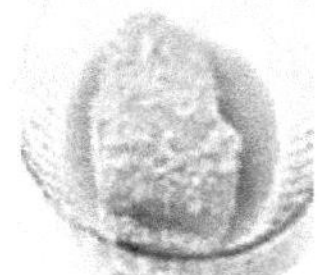

Delicious Spiced Salmon

The combination of herbs in this recipe makes it so yummy.
Total time: 30minutes

Prep time: 10 minutes
Cook time: 20 minutes
Servings: 1
Ingredients:
2 salmon fillets, with skin
1 tsp. fresh lemon juice
1 tsp. extra virgin olive oil
1 clove garlic, sliced
1 tbsp. chopped fresh tarragon
1 tbsp. chopped fresh flat-leaf parsley
3 tbsp. mayonnaise
1 tsp. Dijon mustard
1 pinch cayenne pepper
1/4 tsp. sea salt
Instructions:
1. Properly season the salmon fillet with sea salt as needed, place a foil on a baking sheet and then lightly brush with oil.
2. Set oven broiler on high and place the oven rack about 8" from the heat source.
3. Place the tarragon, garlic and parsley in the bowl of a blender and process in to a loose paste.
4. Combine the mayonnaise, lemon juice, Dijon mustard, and cayenne pepper to the garlic paste and mix well.
5. Place the seasoned salmon fillet in a baking sheet, skin side down and spoon herb mixture over the top and side of each fillet.
6. Cook salmon fillet under heated oven broiler for 5 minutes, put off the broiler and then turn the oven to 350°F
7. Bake for 4 minutes or until fish flake easily with fork. Remove from oven and serve.

Nutrition (per serving): 496 calories, | protein 45.1g, | carbohydrate 2.3g, | fiber 0g, sugar 0g, | fat 33g, | sodium 132.5mg | Potassium: 0mg |

Lemon-Pepper Salmon

This recipe quick and easy to prepare, your entire house hold will love it.
Total time: 30minutes
Prep time: 10 minutes
Cook time: 20 minutes
Servings: 4
Ingredients:
2 tbsp. butter
2 tbsp. extra virgin olive oil
1 tbsp. lemon pepper

4 salmon steaks
1/4 cup water
1 tsp. minced garlic
1 cup chopped fresh tomatoes
1 cup chopped fresh cilantro
2 cups boiling water
1 cup uncooked couscous
1 tsp. sea salt
Instructions:
1. Combine the oil and butter in a large skillet over medium-high heat.
2. Put the salmon in the skillet alongside with lemon pepper, garlic, 1/4 cup of water and salt.
3. Add the cilantro and tomatoes in the skillet, cover and cook until salmon flake easily with fork, for about 15 minutes.
4. Pour 2 cup of water in a cup and let it boil. Pour the hot water to the couscous, cover and let it sit for about 5 minute before serving with salmon, drizzle with sauce from the cooked salmon. Enjoy!
Nutrition (per serving): 498 calories, | protein 31.6g, | carbohydrate 36.2g, | fiber 0g, sugar 0g, | fat 23.5g, | sodium 1038.7mg | Potassium: 0mg |

Spicy Garlic Salmon

This recipe is extraordinarily yummy and can be prepared within a few minutes
Total time: 25minutes
Prep time: 10 minutes
Cook time: 15 minutes
Servings: 2
Ingredients:
1 dried red Chile pepper
2 fillets salmon
2 cloves garlic, finely crushed
1 tbsp. extra virgin olive oil
1 tsp. whole grain mustard
2 tbsp. fresh lime juice
Sea salt and freshly ground black pepper to taste
Instructions:
1. Preheat the oven to 400°F, place aluminum foil in a medium baking dish and coat lightly with cooking spray.
2. Combine the garlic, oil and Chile pepper in the mortar and grind with pestle.
3. Add the lime juice, mustard, salt, and pepper to the mortar and mix until thick paste is formed.

4. Place the fish in the prepared baking dish and coat well with the mixture and bake until it flake easily with a fork, for about 15 minutes.
5. Remove from heat and serve. Enjoy.
Nutrition (per serving): 345 calories, | protein 29.5g, | carbohydrate 3.4g, | fiber 0g, sugar 0g, | fat 23g, | sodium 561.1mg | Potassium: 0mg |

Lemony Orzo with Baked Salmon and Basil Bacon Peas

This recipe is easy and quick to prepare. Your whole family will like
Total time 50minutes
Prep time: 20 minutes
Cook time: 30 minutes
Servings: 4
Ingredients:
1 cup orzo
2 tsp. garlic powder
5 large basil leaves, finely sliced and divided into two
1 1/2 Ib. skin-on, sockeye salmon
1/4 cup butter, melted, divided into two
3 slices bacon, chopped
2 lemons juiced, divided into two
2 tsp. sea salt, divided into two
Freshly ground black pepper to taste
Instructions:
1. Preheat the oven to 450°F, place aluminum foil on a baking dish
2. Pour water in a large pot add a little salt and bring to a boil over medium-high heat. Add the orzo to the pot, cook and stir but not often. Cook the orzo for about 10 minutes or until tender but firm if bite.
3. In a small bowl, combine the garlic powder, 4 basil leaves, and 1/2 tsp. of salt and mix well.
4. Place the salmon fish in the baking dish and let the skin side down and properly brush well with 1 tbsp. of butter and then sprinkle the garlic powder mixture over the salmon fish.
5. Place in the oven and bake for 8 minutes or until fish flake easily with fork. Remove from oven and let rest.
6. In a medium skillet over medium-high heat, place bacon, cook and stir often for about 4 minutes or until bacon turns crispy.
7. Add 1/2 tsp. salt and peas to the bacon skillet, cook and stir for 4 minutes.
8. Combine the remaining lemon juice, 3 tbsp. of butter, 1 tsp.of salt in a small mixing bowl and whisk well.

9. Pour the mixture over the cooked orzo and toss to coat, properly season with salt pepper to taste.

10. Properly divide the coated orzo equally among 4 serving plates and top each plate with salmon and then place the peas on the side.

11. Garnish with rest of the basil leave and drizzle with the remaining lemon juice. Serve and enjoy!

Nutrition (per serving): 702 calories, | protein 51.1g, | carbohydrate 59.7g, | fiber 0g, sugar 0g, | fat 30.1g, | sodium 1278.2mg | Potassium: 0mg |

Yummy Grilled Salmon

Marinate the salmon fillets for at least 6 hour before grilling.

Total time 6 hours 30minutes

Prep time: 10 minutes

Cook time: 20 minutes

Servings: 4

Ingredients:

4 fillets salmon

2 tbsp. soy sauce

1/4 cup extra virgin olive oil

2 tbsp. Balsamic vinegar

2 tbsp. finely sliced green onion

2/3 tsp. Ground ginger

1 1/2 tsp. brown sugar

1 clove garlic, minced

1/2 tsp. crushed red pepper flakes

1/2 tsp. avocado oil

1/8 tsp. salt

Instructions:

1. Combine the olive oil, balsamic vinegar, green onions, brown sugar, red chile flakes, ginger avocado oil, soy sauce and salt in a medium mixing bowl and whisk well.

2. Put the salmon fillet in a glass dish and pour mixture over the fish, cover dish with a plastic wrap and then place in the fridge for at least 6 hours

3. Preheat the gas grill, properly oil the rack and then adjust the height to at least 5 inches coals.

4. Remove the glass dish from the fridge and remove the salmon fillet from the marinade and then place on the grill rack.

5. Grill salmon for 20 minutes and turn once halfway through cooking or until fish flake easily with fork.

6. Remove from heat and enjoy!

Nutrition (per serving): 233 calories, | protein 15.3 g, | carbohydrate 2.9g, | fiber 0g, sugar 0g, | fat 17.6g, | sodium 395.3mg | Potassium: 0mg |

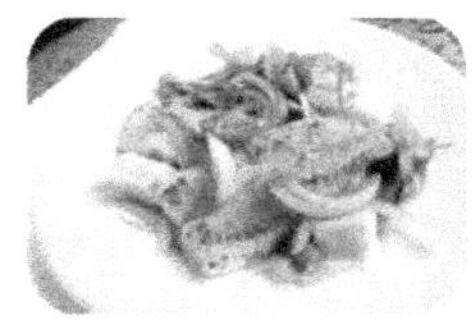

Curry Salmon with Mango

Make this curry salmon with mango within 30 minutes and serve right away
Total time 35minutes
Prep time: 15minutes
Cook time: 20 minutes
Servings: 4

Ingredients:
1 salmon fillet
1/4 cup avocado oil
1 tsp. curry powder
1/4 cup diced red onion
1 small bunch cilantro leaves
1 mango - peeled, removes seed and diced
1 small serrano pepper, diced
1 lime
Sea salt to taste

Instructions:
1. Preheat the oven to 400°F and place aluminum foil on a baking dish
2. Place salmon on the baking dish and fold the aluminum edges over the salmon fish and then crimp to real.
3. Place the baking dish in the oven and bake for 15 minutes or until fish flake easily with fork
4. In a small bowl, combine the curry powder, avocado oil and salt and mix well. Pour the curry powder mixture into the salmon fish.
5. Add the diced mango, Serrano pepper and red onion over the salmon fish
6. To serve garnish with squeeze of lime and cilantro and enjoy.

Nutrition (per serving): 330 calories, | protein 25g, | carbohydrate 12.2g, | fiber 0g, sugar 0g, | fat 20.6g, | sodium 321mg | Potassium: 0mg |

Spicy Citrus Shrimp Salad

Prepare this spicy citrus shrimp salad in less than 30 minutes! Your whole family will love it.

Total time: 20minutes
Prep time: 10 minutes
Cook time: 0 minutes
Servings: 3
Ingredients:
4 cups kale,
1 grapefruit, cut into segments
1 orange, cut into segments
1 blood orange, cut into segments
1/2 small red onion, sliced thin
For the Spicy Shrimp
15-20 shrimp, peeled and vein removed
1/2 tsp. paprika
Tsp. Extra-virgin olive oil
1/2 tsp. chili powder
1/2 tsp. garlic granules
1/2tsp. cumin
1/2 cup fresh grapefruit juice
4 tsp. fine sea salt
For the Grapefruit Vinaigrette
1 tsp. Freshly grated ginger
1 tsp. honey
1 tsp. Dijon mustard
2 tbsp. extra-virgin olive oil
Pinch fine sea salt
Instructions:
1. Place the kale in a medium bowl and add the grapefruit, orange blood orange segments to the bowl.
2. Add the slice onion and put aside.
3. Place the shrimp in a large bowl, add the spices and toss with oil
4. Heat oil in a medium-high heat and add the spiced shrimps.
5. Cook shrimp for 4 minutes, toss and cook for another 4 minutes or until shrimp turns pink and opaque. Transfer to a serving plate and let cool.
6. To make the dressing, combine the dressing ingredients in a small bowl and whisk well. Set aside,
7. To serve, add the salad in a serving plate top with the shrimp and drizzle with the dressing and toss. Enjoy!

Nutrition (per serving): 337 calories, | protein 23g, | carbohydrate 29g, | fiber 4g, sugar 21g, | fat 14g, | sodium 348mg | Potassium: 0mg |

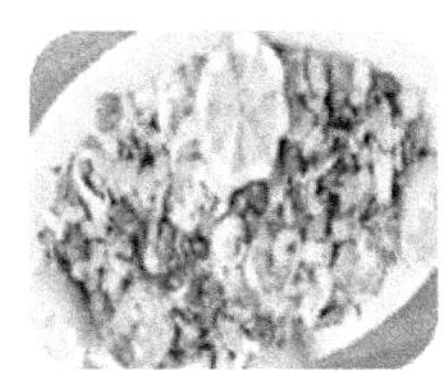

Avocado Shrimp Salad Wraps with Sweet Potato Chips

This recipe is packed with nutrients and very low in carb. You have to bake the potato chips in batches.

Total time: 50 minutes
Prep time: 20 minutes
Cook time: 30 minutes
Servings: 4

Ingredients:
Cooking spray
2 -3 medium sweet potatoes
1/4 small red onion, thinly diced
3/4 pound shrimp (peeled & deveined)
1 1/2 cup grape tomatoes, halved
2 avocados, diced
2 large heads butter head or romaine lettuce
4 fresh basil leaves, thinly sliced
Juice of 2 medium lemons
2 cloves garlic, minced
3 fresh basil leaves, thinly sliced
2 tbsp. white wine vinegar
3 tbsp. avocado oil
1/2 tsp. paprika
Salt to taste
Freshly ground black pepper to taste

Instructions:
1. Preheat the oven to 375°and properly coat the baking sheet with the cooking spray
2. Slice the potato into 1/8 inch thick coins shape and arrange them in the coated baking sheet in an even layer and season with salt and pepper.
3. Roast for 20 minutes and then flip and roast for another 10 minutes or until ready. Remove from heat and let cool.
4. While the last batch of the potato chips is cooking, coat a large skillet with cooking spray and heat over medium heat.
5. Add the shrimp and cook for 2 minutes on both side until shrimp turns pink, stir occasionally. Remove from heat and let cool

6. In a small bowl, combine the lemon juice, avocado oil, vinegar garlic, basil, paprika, salt and pepper and whisk well.
7. Combine the avocados, tomatoes, basil and onion in a large mixing bowl. Add the shrimp and pour the cream over the shrimp and then toast until well coated.
8. Store the shrimp salad in an air tight container and refrigerate until ready to serve.
9. Serve avocado shrimp salad with lettuce wraps. Enjoy!

Avocado Shrimp salad with grapefruit

Total time: 20 minutes
Prep time: 10 minutes
Cook time: 10 minutes
Servings: 2
Ingredients:
1 cup shrimp
2 Tbsp. extra virgin olive oil
1 avocado, cubed
1 grapefruit, cubed
1/4 cup balsamic reduction
1 cup cooked rice, cold
1/2 tsp. sea salt
1/2 tsp. freshly ground pepper

Instructions:
1. Heat the oil in a saucepan over medium-high heat, add the shrimp and cook until pink and opaque.
2. Remove the shrimp from heat and add salt and pepper.
3. Gently pack 1/2 of the cubed avocado as tightly as possible and place at the bottom of a cylinder cup and cover with 1/2 cup rice and then gently pack down.
4. Invert the cylinder cup into a plate and then top with the shrimp, a layer of grapefruit and drizzle with balsamic reduction.
5. Serve right away. Enjoy!
Nutrition (per serving): 393 calories, | protein 14.2g, | carbohydrate 44.7g, | fiber 4.4g, sugar 4.5g, | fat 17.9g, | sodium 109mg | Potassium: 0mg |

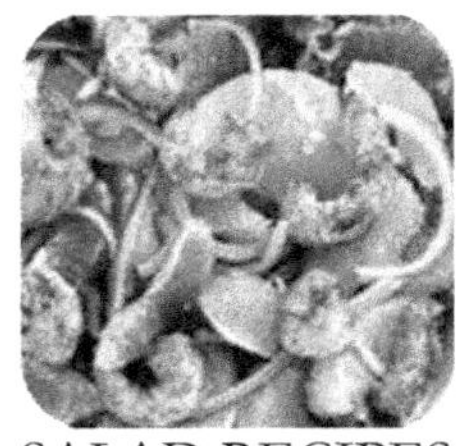

SALAD RECIPES

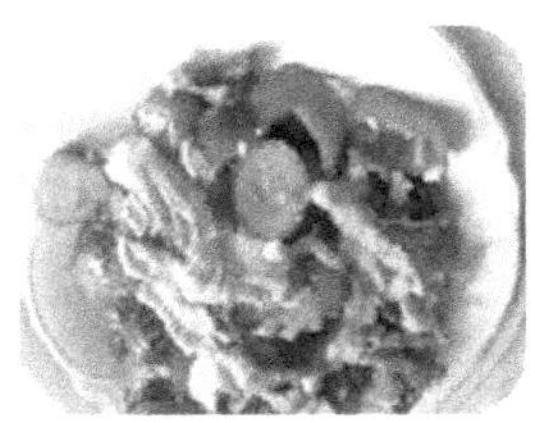

Red Grapefruit Salad with Avocado and Pistachios

This recipe is quick and easy to prepare, it is dairy free, gluten free, low in sodium and packed with nutrient.

Total time: 20minutes

Prep time: 30 minutes

Cook time: 3 0 minutes

Servings: 6

Ingredients:

3 large red grapefruit

1 tbsp. shallot, finely chopped

3 tbsp. extra-virgin olive oil

2 tbsp. white balsamic vinegar

1 tsp. honey

1 tsp. Dijon mustard

1/4 tsp. kosher salt

Freshly ground black pepper

2 firm ripe avocados, finely chopped

1/3 cup unsalted roasted shelled pistachios

1/4 cup fresh chervil

Instructions:

1. With a sharp kitchen knife, remove skin white pith from the grapefruit and through away. Cut each grapefruit into half inch round thick.

2. In a medium mixing bowl, combine shallot, vinegar, honey and mustard and whisk well.

3. Slowly add oil in as you whisk continuously until well combined.

4. Season with sea salt and pepper to taste.

5. In a serving plate, assemble the avocado slices, grapefruit   slices, pistachios and chervil. Drizzle with dressing. Enjoy!

Nutrition (per serving): 272 calories, | protein 3.8g, | carbohydrate 23g, | fiber 32g, sugar7. 2g, |fat 11.3g, | sodium 577.3mg |Potassium: 39.3mg |

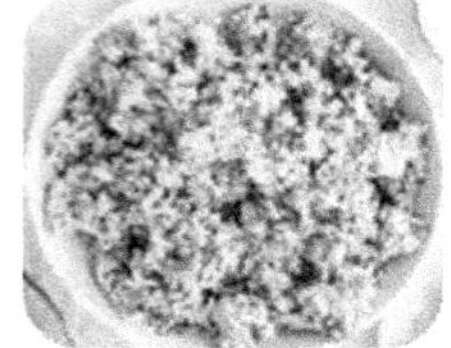

Tuna Salad with Dijon Mustard Vinaigrette

This recipe is loaded with lot of crunchy veggies and herbs make it in less than 20 minutes

Total time: 15 minutes

Prep time: 15 minutes

Cook time: 0 minutes

Servings: 6

Ingredients:

For the Zesty Dijon Mustard Dressing

1 1/2 limes, juice

1 lime zest

1/2 cup Early Harvest extra virgin olive oil

1/2 tsp. sumac

2 1/2 tsp. good quality Dijon mustard

Pinch of salt and pepper

For the Tuna Salad

3 cans tuna, 5 ounces each (use quality tuna of your choice)

1/2 English cucumber, finely chopped

2 1/2 celery stalks, finely chopped

4-5 whole small radishes, stems removed, chopped

1/2 cup pitted Kalamata olives, halved

1/2 medium-sized red onion, finely chopped

3 green onions, both white and green parts, chopped

1 cup chopped fresh parsley, stems removed,

1/2 cup finely chopped fresh mint leaves, stems removed

Homemade Pita chips for serving

6 slices heirloom tomatoes for serving

Instructions:

1. Combine the Dijon mustard, lime juice and lime zest in a small mixing bowl and whisk.
2. Add the sumac, oil, salt and pepper and whisk until well mixed and smooth. Set aside.
3. Combine the tuna, chopped veggies, parsley, olives and mint leaves in a large mixing bowl and mix well with a spoon.
4. Add the dressing to the salad and mix until salad is well coated. Cover the bowl with a lid and put in the fridge for 30 minutes before serving.
5. To serve, divide salad among 6 serving plate and top with pita chips and each plate with a slice of heirloom tomatoes on the side. Enjoy! You can also serve salad in a pita pocket for a sandwich.
Nutrition (per serving): 299 calories, | protein 25.7g, | carbohydrate 6.6g, | fiber 0g, sugar 2.7g, | fat 19.2g, | sodium 126.1mg | Potassium: 0mg |

Thai Crab Salad with Creamy Coconut-Lime Dressing

Delicious salad and dressing to enjoy with family and friends
Total time: 25 minutes
Prep time: 25 minutes
Cook time: 0 minutes
Servings: 2
Ingredients:
1/2 cup full-fat coconut milk
1/2 tsp. dried crushed chili
1 1/2 tbsp. lime juice
2 cups cabbage finely sliced
1 tsp. sugar
1 cup fresh coriander leaves, lightly
3 tbsp. fish sauce
3 green onions, finely sliced
2 cups bean sprouts
1/3 cup dry roasted peanuts or cashews finely chopped
1 carrot, grated
1 cup prepared crab meat, freshly-cooked, canned and frozen
Instructions:
1. Combine the coconut milk, chili flakes, lime juice, fish sauce and sugar in a cup and stir until well mixed. Set aside.
2. Place the sliced cabbage in a bowl, add the rest of the veggies and set aside 1/2 of the coriander.
3. Add the crab meat. Stir the dressing again, drizzle over the salad an f then toss well to combine.
4. Taste and adjust as needed.

5. Dived among two serving plate and top with reserved coriander and nuts. Serve immediately or chilled. Enjoy!
Nutrition (per serving): 453 calories, | protein 34g, | carbohydrate 11g, | fiber 1g, sugar 0g, | fat 8g, | sodium 0mg | Potassium: 0mg |

Berry-Beet Salad

This salad is packed with flavor and taste so yummy.
Total time: 50 minutes
Prep time: 20 minutes
Cook time: 30 minutes
Servings: 4
Ingredients:
1 each fresh golden and red beets
1/4 cup balsamic vinegar
2 tbsp. walnut oil
1/2 cup sliced fresh strawberries
1/2 cup fresh raspberries
1/2 cup fresh blackberries
1 shallot, thinly sliced
3 tbsp. chopped walnuts, toasted
1 tbsp. fresh basil, thinly sliced
1 tsp. honey
4 cups torn mixed salad greens
1 oz. crumbled feta
Dash of salt
Dash of pepper
Instructions:
1. Preheat the oven to 400F°
2. In an 8 inches square baking pan, place the beets. Add water to the beets, cover and bake until softened, about for 30 minutes.
3. Combine the honey, vinegar, walnut oil, salt and pepper in a small bowl and whisk well. Set aside.
4. Remove the beets from the oven and let it cool before peeling and slicing.
5. Combine the beets, berries, shallot and toasted walnuts in a large bowl.
6. Pour the dressing over the mixture and gently toss until coated.
7. Divide the salad greens into 4 serving plates and with the beet mixture and then sprinkle with crumbled feta and basil.
Nutrition (per serving): 183calories, | protein 4 g, | carbohydrate 18g, | fiber 5g, sugar 11g, | fat 12g, | sodium 124mg | Potassium: 0mg |

Egg Chickpea salad

This egg chickpea salad is satisfying and packed with flavor and texture. Can be ready in less than 20 minutes

Total time: 15 minutes

Prep time: 15 minutes

Cook time: 0 minutes

Servings: 8

Ingredients:

2 1/2 tsp. Dijon mustard

1 large lemon, zested and juiced

1 tsp. sumac

1/3 cup extra virgin olive oil

1/2 tsp. coriander

1 garlic clove, minced

1/2 tsp. cayenne pepper

Sea Salt to taste

Freshly ground black pepper to taste

For Salad

2 cans chickpeas, rinsed and drained

5 large hard boiled eggs, sliced

2 celery ribs, finely chopped

2 English cucumbers, diced

2 -3 green onions, trimmed, and chopped

1/2 cup shredded red cabbage

1/2 cup packed chopped fresh parsley leaves

1/2 cup packed chopped fresh mint leaves

Instructions:

1. Combine all the ingredients for the dressing in small mixing bowl and mix well. Set aside.

2. Combine all the ingredients for salad in a large mixing bowl, except the eggs, pour the dressing into salad and mix well.

3. Add the sliced egg to the bowl and gently mix. Taste the salad and add more salt and pepper if needed.

4. Sprinkle a little more of sumac and set aside for about 10 minutes or more before serving. Enjoy!

Nutrition (per serving): 193 calories, | protein 7.9g, | carbohydrate 12.9g, | fiber 9.6g, sugar 2.6g, | fat 12.9g, | sodium 52.4mg | Potassium: 0mg |

Shredded Carrot Salad

A quick put together salad for busy people.

Total time: 5 minutes

Prep time: 5 minutes

Cook time: 0 minutes
Servings: 5
Ingredients:
7 carrots (wash, peeled & shredded)
3 tbsp. olive oil
1/2 tsp. Dijon mustard
1 tbsp. lemon juice
1/4 tsp. salt
1/8 tsp. freshly ground black pepper
Instructions:
1. Combine the mustard, lemon juice, and oil in a small bowl and whisk until well mixed.
2. Drizzle the dressing into the shredded carrots and sprinkle with salt and pepper and
 Toss well.
3. Place the salad in the fridge and chill for 30 minutes before serving. Enjoy!
Nutrition (per serving): 232 calories, | protein 1g, | carbohydrate 13g, | fiber 0g, sugar 0g, |fat 21g, | sodium 0mg | Potassium: 0mg |

Moroccan Carrot Salad

This Moroccan carrot is colorful and flavorful
Total time: 23 minutes
Prep time: 15 minutes
Cook time: 8 minutes
Servings: 4
Ingredients:
7 carrots (washed, peeled, and cut into rounds)
3 tbsp. freshly squeezed lemon juice
2 tbsp. olive oil
1/2 tsp. cumin
2 cloves garlic (peeled and chopped)
1/2 tsp. paprika
2 cups of water
Kosher salt to taste
Freshly ground pepper to taste
Instructions:
1. Pour 2 cups of water in a saucepan, add salt and bring to a boil over a medium high heat.
2. Reduce heat to low heat, add the carrot and simmer until carrot is softened, for about 8 minutes

3. Drain the carrots in a colander and rinse under running water and then transfer to a bowl.
4. Combine the lemon juice, cumin, olive oil, garlic, and paprika in a small bowl and whisk well.
5. Drizzle the dressing over the carrot and toss well. Add salt and pepper to taste.
6. Serve salad immediately or place in the fridge to chill for 30 minutes before serving.
Nutrition (per serving): 203calories, | protein 4g, | carbohydrate 33g, | fiber 0g, sugar 0g, | fat 8g, | sodium 0mg | Potassium: 0mg |

Greek Stuffed Avocado

This salad recipe is light and satisfying. it's quick and easy to put together
Total time: 15 minutes
Prep time: 15 minutes
Cook time: 0 minutes
Servings: 3
Ingredients:
2 avocados, halved and pitted
8 cherry tomatoes, halved
2 tbsp. black olives, roughly
2 tbsp. finely chopped red onion
1/2 Persian cucumber, cubed
1/4 cup feta, cubed
2 tsp. coarsely chopped fresh dill
2 tbsp. avocado oil
1 tbsp. lemon juice
Salt and pepper to taste
Instructions:
1. Combine the tomatoes, olives, cucumber, red onion, feta, lemon juice, oil, and dill in a bowl and toss
2. Season well with salt and pepper to taste.
3. Scoop out the flash of each avocado half and leave half inch border.
4. Chop the flash of avocado you scoop out into small sizes and stir into the salad mixture.
5. Fill each avocado half with the salad and serve. Enjoy!

Tomato and Avocado Salad

This tomato and avocado salad is packed with flavor; you can enjoy it with chips if you want.
Total time: 15 minutes
Prep time: 15 minutes

Cook time: 0 minutes
Servings: 4
Ingredients:
1/4 cup avocado oil
3 avocados, cubed
1 lemon juice
1/4 tsp. cumin
1 pack cherry tomatoes, halved
1 small cucumber, sliced into half moons
1/3 cup corn
2 tbsp. chopped cilantro
Salt and pepper to taste
Instructions:
1. Combine the lime juice, avocado oil, and cumin a small bowl and whisk well, season with salt and pepper.
2. Combine the tomatoes, avocados, cucumber, cilantro and corn in a large bowl, add the dressing and toss gently. Serve and enjoy immediately.
5. To serve, top with diced tomato and enjoy immediately.

Broccoli Salad with Greek yogurt

This broccoli salad recipe is satisfying packed with nutrient.
Total time: 10 minutes
Prep time: 10 minutes
Cook time: 0 minutes
Servings: 6
Ingredients:
1/4 cup nonfat Greek yogurt
5 cups chopped broccoli (stems removed and cut in florets)
2 tbsp. Balsamic vinaigrette
2 tbsp. roasted and salted sunflower seeds
1/4 cup raisins
1/4 teaspoon kosher salt
1/4 teaspoon freshly ground black pepper
Instructions:
1. Combine Greek yogurt and vinaigrette in a mixing bowl and whisk until very smooth.
2. Add a little water (about 1 tbsp.) to thin out the mixture, season the mixture with 1/4 tsp. salt and pepper. Set aside.
3. Combine sunflower seeds broccoli, and raisins in a large mixing bowl, top with the dressing and toss well to coat.
4. Refrigerate for 30minutes or more before serving. Enjoy!

Nutrition (per serving): 86 calories, | protein 3g, | carbohydrate 12g, | fiber 2g, sugar 0g, | fat 3g, | sodium 1225mg | Potassium: 0mg |

Broccoli Salad

This broccoli salad is loaded with flavor and nutrient. Your entire house hold will love it.
Total time: 40 minutes
Prep time: 20 minutes
Cook time: 20 minutes
Servings: 6
Ingredients:
5 cups chopped broccoli (stems removed and cut in florets)
5 bacon strips low sodium
1/2 cup dried cranberries unsweetened
1/2 cup sunflower seeds
1/4 cup red onion diced
1/2 cup plain yogurt
1/4 cup cheddar cheese coarsely grated
1/4 cup quality mayo (I use avocado oil)
Freshly ground black pepper to taste
Instructions:
1. Preheat the oven to 400°F. Place unbleached parchment paper on a large baking sheet.
2. Place bacon strips on the baking sheet and bake until crispy, for 20 minutes. When is done cooking transfer to triple folded paper towel to drain the fat.
3. Cut the broccoli florets into small sizes and place a salad bowl, add sunflower seeds, red onion, dried cranberries and cheese to the bowl.
4. Combine yogurt and mayo in a bowl and whisk well, crumble the bacon.
5. Add the dressing to the crumbled bacon, stir well and then set aside to sit.
6. Refrigerate for 30 minutes or more before serving, you can also serve immediately if you want.
Note: save the leftover in the fridge for up to 3 days
Nutrition (per serving): 264 calories, | protein 9g, | carbohydrate 20g, | fiber 4g, sugar 10g, | fat 18g, | sodium 265mg | Potassium: 0mg |

Greek Salad with Edamame

This recipe is packed with nutrients and refreshing. It takes only 20 minutes to be ready.
Total time: 20 minutes
Prep time: 30 minutes
Cook time: 0 minutes
Servings: 4

Ingredients:
1/4 cup red-wine vinegar
3 tbsp. extra-virgin olive oil
8 cups chopped romaine
3 cup frozen shelled edamame, thawed
1/2 European cucumber, sliced
1 cup halved cherry or grape tomatoes
1/2 cup crumbled feta cheese
1/4 cup slivered red onion
1/4 cup slivered fresh basil
1/4 cup sliced Kalamata olives
1/4 tsp. salt
1/4 tsp. black ground pepper
Instructions:
1. Combine the oil, vinegar, salt and pepper in a large mixing bowl and whisk well.
2. Add edamame, tomatoes, basil, romaine, cucumber, olives feta, and onion to the bowl and toss until well coated.
3. Serve and enjoy.
Nutrition (per serving): 344 calories, | protein 17.1g, | carbohydrate 19.9g, | fiber 8.8g, sugar 6.3g, | fat 23.3g, | sodium 488.7mg | Potassium: 907.6mg |

Broccoli, Apple & Walnuts Salad

Total time: 25 minutes
Prep time: 20 minutes
Cook time: 5 minutes
Servings: 6
Ingredients:
2 medium heads of broccoli, chopped
2 tbsp. lemon juice
1 apple, cored and finely chopped
1/2 cup walnuts, coarsely chopped
1 large carrot, grated
1/4 cup dried cranberries
1 cup mayonnaise
1/4 cup onion, finely chopped
1 garlic clove, finely minced
Sea salt and freshly ground black pepper to taste
Instructions:
1. Combine the broccoli, apple, walnuts, carrot, dried cranberries, onion, salt and pepper to taste in a large mixing bowl and mix well.

2. In a small mixing bowl, add the mayonnaise, garlic and lemon juice and whisk well.

3. Add dressing as needed to the salad and toss well to combine.

4. Refrigerate for 30 minutes or more before serving, you can serve immediately if you want. Enjoy!

Nutrition (per serving): 126 calories, | protein 5g, | carbohydrate 25g, | fiber 0g, sugar 50g, | fat 50g, | sodium 183mg | Potassium: 0mg |

Quinoa Chickpea Salad with Roasted Red Pepper Hummus Dressing

This salad recipe is packed with flavor and it is perfect with the dressing. It is high in fiber.

Total time: 10 minutes

Prep time: 10 minutes

Cook time: 0 minutes

Servings: 1

Ingredients:

2 tbsp. hummus, original or roasted red pepper flavor

1 tbsp. unsalted sunflower seeds

2 cups mixed salad greens

1 tbsp. Lemon juice

1 tbsp. Chopped roasted red pepper

1/2 cup cooked quinoa

1 tbsp. chopped fresh parsley

1/2 cup chickpeas, rinsed

Pinch of salt

Pinch of ground pepper

Instructions:

1. Combine the lemon juice, hummus and red pepper in a small plate and stir well. Add little water as needed.

2. Assemble the chickpeas, quinoa and greens in a large mixing bowl. Top with parsley, sunflower, salt and pepper.

3. Serve salad with the dressing and enjoy.

Nutrition (per serving): 379 calories, | protein 16g, | carbohydrate 58.5g, | fiber 13.2g, sugar 2.9g, | fat .29.9, | sodium 606.8mg | Potassium: 891.7mg |

DRINK RECIPES

Pumpkin Spice Latte

Total time: 10 minutes
Prep time: 5 minutes
Cook time: 5 minutes
Servings: 1
Ingredients:
1 cup almond milk
2 tbsp. pure pumpkin puree
1/4 cup strong brewed coffee
1/4 tsp. pumpkin pie spice, plus more for sprinkling
1/4 tsp. pure vanilla extract
1 tbsp. Sugar
Sweetened whipped cream, for serving
Instructions:
1. Combine the pumpkin puree, milk, pumpkin pie spice, sugar, and vanilla in a microwave safe bowl, cover the microwave bowl with a plastic wrap and leave a little opening. Microwave for 2 minutes or until milk is hot.
2. Whisk the mixture until foamy, for about 30 seconds.
3. Pour coffee into a mug, add the milk mixture and top with the whipped cream and then sprinkle with the pumpkin pie spice. Enjoy!
Nutrition (per serving): 100 calories, | protein 0g, | carbohydrate 0g, | fiber 0g, sugar 0g, | fat 0g, | sodium 0mg | Potassium: 0mg |

Simple Iced green tea

This iced green tea is perfect for summer and quick to prepare.
Total time: 10 minutes
Prep time: 5 minutes
Cook time: 5 minutes
Servings: 1
Ingredients:
1/4 cup unsweetened Blackberries, frozen,
1 cup almond, unsweetened
1/8 tsp. Cinnamon
1 scoop Quest Vanilla Milkshake Protein Powder
1/2 cup ice cube
1/8 tsp. Allspice
Instructions:
1. Combine all food processor or blender and blend until smooth. Add the ice and pulse for twice.
Transfer to a serving glass cup and serve.
Nutrition (per serving): 180.6calories, | protein 25.5g, | carbohydrate 0g, | fiber 3.1g, sugar 0g, | fat 5.2g, | sodium 0mg | Potassium: 0mg |

Lemon Ginger Green Tea
Total time: 24 hours 5 minutes
Prep time: 5 minutes
Cook time: 0 minute
Servings: 1
Ingredients:
8 green tea bags
1 lemon, sliced
1/2 cup Stevia Sweetener
8 fresh mint leaves
1 cup fresh ginger, peeled and sliced (about 1 cup)
2 quarts water
Instructions:
1. Pour the water in a large pitcher and add the 8 green tea bags, cover the
pitcher and put in the fridge for 24 hours.
2. Take the pitcher out from the fridge and remove from tea bags.
3. Add Stevia Sweetener, ginger, lemon slices and mint to the pitcher and
stir until the sweetener dissolved. Enjoy
*Nutrition (per serving): 20 calories, | protein 1g, | carbohydrate 21g, | fiber 1g, sugar
0g, | fat 0g, | sodium 0mg | Potassium: 0mg |*

Warm Honey Green Tea

This green tea is packed with antioxidants and flavor
Total time: 15 minutes
Prep time: 10 minutes
Cook time: 0minutes
Servings: 4
Ingredients:
4 green tea bags
4 orange peel strips
4 cups water
4 lemon peel strips
4 lemon slices
2 tsp. honey
Instructions:
1. Combine the water, orange peel strips and lemon peel strips in a
saucepan and bring to a boil over medium-high heat.
2. Reduce the heat to low heat and let it simmer uncovered for about 10
minutes. Remove the peels strips with slotted spoon and discard.
3. Add the tea bags in the teapot and then pour into the simmering water
immediately.

4. Cover the pan and let it steep following the package instructions for 3 minutes.
5. Remove the tea bags from the water and squeeze out the liquid gently and throw away the tea bags.
6. Add the honey and stir well. Divide equally among 4 heatproof cups and garnish each cup with lemon slices and enjoy.
Nutrition (per serving): 16 calories, | protein 0.2g, | carbohydrate 0.2g, | fiber 0.6g, sugar 3.2g, |fat 0g, | sodium 7.7mg |Potassium: 109.1mg |

Honeydew Mint Iced Tea

Total time: 60 minutes
Prep time: 10 minutes
Cook time: 12minutes
Servings: 8
Ingredients:
5 Green tea bags
1 cup mint leaf
3 cups cubed peeled honeydew melon about half melon
 1/3 cup granulated sugar
Instructions:
1. Pour 8 cups of boiled water in heatproof bowl and steep in the tea bags for 4 minutes and the discard the tea bags.
2. Combine the melon, mint leave, water and sugar in a saucepan and bring to a boil over medium-high heat.
3. Reduce the heat to low heat and let it simmer for 8 minutes or until the melon is broken. Add the melon to the tea and let it cool for 30 minutes, at room temperature. Place in the fridge for at least 2 hours.
4. Line cheesecloth in a sieve, place on a pitcher and strain, press until beverage remains clear. Enjoy with ice cubes
Nutrition (per serving): 53.0 calories, | protein 0.2g, | carbohydrate 14g, | fiber 0g, sugar 1g, |fat 0g, | sodium 7mg |Potassium: 0mg |

3 ingredients Raspberry Iced Tea

This recipe is so colorful and refreshing
Total time: 60 minutes
Prep time: 10 minutes
Cook time: 12 minutes
Servings: 8
Ingredients:
4 tea bags
1/2 cup granulated sugar
 2 cups raspberries

8 cups boiling water
Instructions:
1. Pour 8 cups of boiled water in heatproof bowl and steep in the tea bags for 4 minutes and the discard the tea bags.
2. Combine the raspberries, 1 cup of water and sugar in a saucepan and bring to a boil over medium heat.
3. Reduce the heat to low heat, simmer and stir until raspberries are tender, remove from heat and add to the tea. Let it cool for 30 minutes at room temperature before place in the fridge for 2 hours.
4. Line cheesecloth in a sieve, place on a pitcher and strain, press until beverage remains clear. Enjoy with ice cubes
Nutrition (per serving): 62.0calories, | protein 0.2g, | carbohydrate 15g, | fiber 0.6g, sugar 1g, |fat 0g, | sodium 8mg | Potassium: 0mg |

Citrus Mint Iced Tea

This recipe is packed with fresh herbs and takes a few minutes to put together.
Total time: 60 minutes
Prep time: 10 minutes
Cook time: 12 minutes
Servings: 6
Ingredients:
6 tea bags
 1/2 cup fresh mint leaves
1/4 cup granulated sugar
 3 lemons
 3 limes, finely sliced
3 oranges
 6 cups boiling water
1 handful ice cubes
Instructions:
1. Combine the tea bags, lemon, mint leaves orange, and lime slices in a teapot, add 6 cups of boiling water and let it steep for 10 minutes
2. Line cheesecloth in a sieve, place on a pitcher and strain, add sugar and stir very well to dissolve the sugar. Enjoy with ice cubes.
Nutrition (per serving): 34 calories, | protein 0g, | carbohydrate 9g, | fiber 0g, sugar 1g, |fat 0g, | sodium 7mg | Potassium: 0mg |

Grapefruit Jalapeño Margarita

This recipe is delicious and refreshing!
Total time: 30minutes
Prep time: 30 minutes
Cook time: 3 0 minutes

Servings: 2
Ingredients:
6 tbsp. tequila
4 tbsp. fresh lime juice
1/2 cup freshly-squeezed grapefruit juice
5 tsp. simple syrup
3 jalapeño slices
ice
For the chili powder-salt mixture:
2 tsp. chili powder
1 lime wedge
2 tbsp.sea salt
Jalapeño slices and Small grapefruit wedges for garnish
Instructions:
1. Put the tequila in a large cup; add the jalapeño together with seeds. Set aside and let it sit for at least 30 minutes.
2. Remove the jalapeño from the cup. Combine chili powder sea salt in a small rimmed plate set aside.
3. Run a lime wedge around the rim of the glasses, dip the rims in the chili powder mixture and then twist to coat.
4. Combine all the margarita ingredients in a cocktail shaker fill with ice cube and then shake until well combined.
5. Transfer to a serving glasses and top with some jalapeno slices and grapefruit wedges. Enjoy!
Nutrition (per serving): 153 calories, | protein 0g, | carbohydrate 12.6g, | fiber 0.8g, sugar 4.4g, | fat 0g, | sodium 6mg | Potassium: 0mg |

Pineapple and Red Grapefruit smoothie

This mix fruit smoothie is packed with nutrient.
Total time: 5 minutes
Prep time: 5 minutes
Cook time: 0 minutes
Servings: 2
Ingredients:
1 1/2 cup orange juice
1 dole red grapefruit sunrise cup
1 cup strawberries, frozen
1 cup vanilla Greek yogurt
1 cup pineapple, frozen
Handful of ice
Instructions:

1. Combine all ingredients in a food processor or blender and blend until smooth.
2. Transfer to a serving cup and enjoy.
Nutrition (per serving): 95 calories, | protein 3.7g, | carbohydrate 18.1g, | fiber 1.3g, sugar 14.7g, | fat 1g, | sodium 36mg | Potassium: 0mg |

Quick Grapefruit Popsicles

Total time: 20 minutes
Prep time: 10 minutes
Cook time: 10 minutes
Servings: 8
Ingredients:
1 cup drinkable water
1 cup sugar
1 tsp. grapefruit zest
2 cups freshly-squeezed ruby red grapefruit juice
2 tsp. Freshly-squeezed lemon juice
Instructions:
1. In a medium saucepan over medium-high heat, add the water, sugar and grapefruit zest and let it boil. Stir often until sugar is fully dissolved.
2. Remove from heat for a while.
3. Add lemon and grapefruit juice and then strain out through a fine-mesh sieve and let cool.
4. Divide the cooled mixture among the 8 Popsicle molds and put in the freezer to freeze for about 4 hours or more. Enjoy!
Nutrition (per serving): 66 calories, | protein 1g, | carbohydrate 17.3g, | fiber 1g, sugar 16.6g, | fat 2g, | sodium 2mg | Potassium: 0mg |

Champagne Grapefruit Mojito

This grapefruit recipe is so easy to prepare, it a perfect mix of sweet and sour, you will love.
Total time: 5 minutes
Prep time: 5 minutes
Cook time: 0 minutes
Servings: 2
Ingredients:
1 Tbsp. agave nectar
12 mint leaves
2 tbsp. lime juice
1 cup ice broken into large cubes
3 oz. rum
1/3 cup champagne club soda

Instructions:

1. Add the grapefruit juice and wedges in a shaker flowed by agave, mint, ice, lime juice and wedges, crush to release flavor.
2. Add the good rum and shake well.
3. Remove the wedges from the mixture (grapefruit and lime wedges)
4. Fill 10 oz. glasses with the broken ice, pour the grapefruit and mint mixture to the glass up to half of the glass.
5. Add the champagne to the glass cup and stir well to combine.
6. Garnish the drink with mint stem and grapefruit wedge. Serve and enjoy.

Nutrition (per serving): 135 calories, | protein 1g, | carbohydrate 9g, | fiber 1g, sugar 7g, | fat 1g, | sodium 9mg | Potassium: 0mg |

DESSERT RECIPES

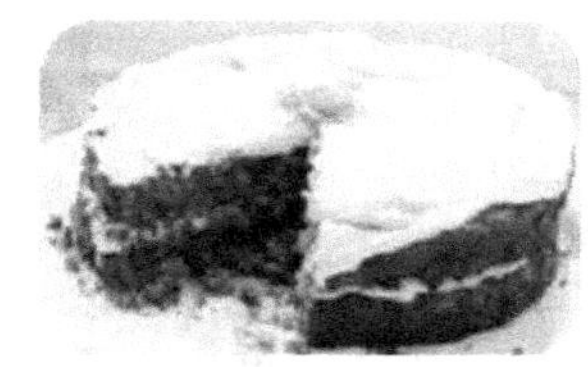

Healthy Apricot Balls with Cashews, Dates and Coconut

Boost your energy with this recipe, it is very easy to put together and so yummy.

Total time: 10 minutes
Prep time: 10 minutes
Cook time: 0 minutes
Servings: 20 balls

Ingredients:

1 cup dried apricots
2 cups cashew nuts, raw, unsalted
1/3 cup shredded unsweetened coconut
1/4 cup chopped dates
1 tsp. orange Zest
1/2 tsp. ground ginger
1 tsp. lemon Zest
1/2 tsp. cinnamon
1/8 tsp. Sea salt

Instructions:

1. In a bowl of food processor, combine the cashew nuts, apricots, coconut and dates and process until crumbly
2. Add lemon zest, orange zest, spices and salt to the mixture and process until well combined. Set the food processor on high and process again until mixture start to stick.
3. Place a parchment paper on a tray and shape the mixture into 20 1 inch balls
4. store in an air tight container and place in the freezer for up to 3 weeks or in fridge for up to 3 days.
Nutrition (per serving): 102 calories, | protein 2g, | carbohydrate 9g, | fiber 1g, sugar 5g, | fat 4g, | sodium 17mg | Potassium: 0mg |

Lemon Olive Oil Cake

This recipe is packed with whole, unprocessed ingredients and very easy to prepare.
Total time: 55 minutes
Prep time: 10 minutes
Cook time: 45 minutes
Servings: 8
Ingredients:
2 cups whole wheat pastry flour
1 cup unsweetened almond milk
1/3 cup olive oil
1 tbsp. lemon zest
1 tbsp. lemon juice
3/4 cup turbinado sugar
1 tsp. baking soda
1/2 tsp. Salt
For the glaze:
1 cup powdered sugar
1/2 tsp. vanilla extract
1-2 tbsp. lemon juice
Instructions:
1. Preheat the oven to 350°F. Place a parchment paper in a 9 inches baking pan and properly coat with a nonstick cooking spray.
2. Combine the milk, 1 tbsp. of lemon juice and lemon zest in a bowl and set aside for about 5 minutes.
3. Combine the oil and sugar in a large bowl and whisk until smooth and creamy. Add the buttermilk mixture and whisk well.
4. Combine the flour, baking soda and salt in medium bowl and add the buttermilk mixture and stir well.
5. Transfer batter in the prepared baking pan and smooth the top. Place the pan in the oven and for 45 minutes.

6. Remove the pan from the oven and let cool for 10 minutes in the pan before removing to a cooling rack and set over a baking sheet to cool off.
7. Meanwhile, combine the lemon juice, vanilla and sugar in a bowl and whisk until smooth.
8. Pour the glaze over the cooled cake and let any excess trip off the cake onto the baking sheet beneath.
Nutrition (per serving): 321 calories, | protein 4g, | carbohydrate 56g, | fiber 3g, sugar 34g, | fat 4g, | sodium 325mg | Potassium: 0mg |

Yummy Spanish Oatmeal Bowls

 Total time: 30 minutes
Prep time: 15 minutes
Cook time: 15 minutes
Servings: 4
Ingredients:
Oatmeal
1 cup old fashioned oats
2 cups almond milk
1/2 tsp. salt, divided
1/4 tsp pepper
Chorizo
1/2 tbsp. olive oil
1/2 onion, chopped
2 cloves garlic, finely chopped
Sauce and toppings
1/3 cup roughly chopped roasted red peppers
1/2 pound uncooked chorizo
1 tbsp. tomato paste
1 clove garlic
1 tbsp. red wine vinegar
1/2 tap. Smoked paprika
Pinch of cayenne
1/4 cup toasted almonds
2 poached eggs
Fresh chopped parsley
Instructions:
1. In a saucepan, combine the oatmeal, milk, 1/4 tsp. of salt and pepper and let boil over medium-high heat.
2. Reduce the heat low heat and let it simmer, stir but not often.
3. In a skillet over medium heat, heat oil and add onion, sprinkle with 1/4 tsp. of salt and let it simmer for 3 minutes.

4. Add the garlic to the skillet and cook for 1 minute more. Add the chorizo and make sure you it up into pieces a spoon and then let it cook for 5 minutes. Remove the skillet from the heat.
5. Combine the red peppers, garlic, tomato paste, paprika, cayenne, almonds and vinegar in a food processor and process until chunky and pasty.
6. Evenly place oatmeal into a 4 serving bowl and top with 2 tbsp. of romesco sauce, 1/4 cup of chorizo mixture and 1 poached egg. Sprinkle with fresh chopped parsley. Serve and enjoy.
Nutrition (per serving): 435 calories, | protein 6.2g, | carbohydrate 43.3g, | fiber 6.2g, sugar 19.7g, | fat 4g, | sodium 573mg | Potassium: 0mg |

Mixed Berries Balsamic with Honey Yogurt

Total time: 15 minutes
Prep time: 15 minutes
Cook time: 0 minutes
Servings: 4
Ingredients:
1 1/2 cups strawberries, hulled and halved
1 cup raspberries
2/3 cup whole-milk plain Greek yogurt
1 cup blueberries
1 tbsp. balsamic vinegar
2 tsp. honey
Instructions:
1. Combine the blueberries, strawberries, raspberries and balsamic vinegar in a large bowl and toss well. Let the mixture sit for at least 10 minutes.
2. Combine the honey and yogurt in s small bowl and stir well.
3. Divide the berries equally among 4 serving bowls and top each bowl with a dollop of honey and yogurt mixture. Enjoy!
Nutrition (per serving): 111 calories, | protein 4g, | carbohydrate 18.6g, | fiber 4g, sugar 12.9g, | fat 3g, | sodium 24.7mg | Potassium: 0mg |

Caprese Avocado Toast

Total time: 15 minutes
Prep time: 15 minutes
Cook time: 0 minutes
Servings: 2
Ingredients:
2 slices whole-wheat bread
1 medium avocado, halved and pit removed
8 grape tomatoes, halved

2 tbsp. balsamic glaze
12 bite-sized mozzarella balls
4 large fresh basil leaves, torn
Instructions:
1. Toast the 2 whole-wheat bread and mash the avocado in a bowl as the
bread is toasting.
2. When the bread is done toasting, spread the mashed avocado on the
toast bread and top each slices with mozzarella balls, tomatoes and basil
leaves,
3 Drizzle each slice with balsamic glaze and enjoy!
*Nutrition (per serving): 649 calories, | protein 23.9g, | carbohydrate 86.4g, | fiber
10.5g, sugar 11g, | fat 24.6g, | sodium 1028.3mg | Potassium: 0mg |*

Easy and yummy Muesli

Total time: 30 minutes
Prep time: 15 minutes
Cook time: 15 minutes
Servings: 8
Ingredients:
1/2 cup sliced almonds
3 1/2 cups rolled oats
1/2 cup wheat bran
1/2 tsp. ground cinnamon
1/4 cup dried apricots, coarsely chopped
1/4 cup raw pecans, coarsely chopped
1/4 cup raw pepitas shelled pumpkin seeds
1/2 cup unsweetened coconut flakes
1/4 cup dried cherries
1/2 tsp. sea salt
Instructions:
1. Combine the nuts, grains and seeds in a skillet and toast over medium
heat.
2. Arrange 2 racks to divide the oven into thirds and then preheat the oven
to 350°F
3. Combine the wheat brain, oats, cinnamon and salt in a rimmed baking
sheet and toast well to combine. Spread the oats mixture into an even layer.
4. Transfer to the oven and place oats on top of the rack and place the nuts
on the bottom and bake for about 12 minutes. Add the coconut.
5. Remove the baking sheet with the nuts and set put aside to cool to room
temperature.

6. Sprinkle the coconut over the oats and place back to the oven and bake for 5 minutes or until coconuts turns golden brown. Remove from oven and put aside to cool for 10 minutes

7. Transfer to the both baking sheet contents in a large bowl and add apricots, dried fruit and cherries and toss well to combine.

8. Transfer to an airtight container and store at room temperature for up to a month.

9. Transfer to an airtight container. Muesli can be stored in an airtight container at room temperature for up to 1 month.

10. To serve, top with fresh fruit and drizzle with honey and enjoy or as desired.

Nutrition (per serving): 275 calories, | protein 8.5g, | carbohydrate 36.5g, | fiber 7.5g, sugar 6.9g, | fat 13.0g, | sodium 122.5mg | Potassium: 0mg |

Goat Cheese and Kale Frittata cup

Total time: 50 minutes
Prep time: 15 minutes
Cook time: 35 minutes
Servings: 8
Ingredients:
2 cups chopped lacinato kale, remove the leaves from the kale ribs, Wash and dry and then cut into 1/2-inch-wide strips.
1 garlic clove, thinly sliced
8 large eggs
3 tbsp. extra virgin olive oil
1/4 tsp. red pepper flakes
1/2 tsp. dried thyme
1/4 cup goat cheese, crumbled
1/4 tsp. sea salt
Dash ground black pepper
Instructions:
1. Preheat the oven to 350°F.
2. Heat 1 tbsp. of oil in a 10 inches nonstick skillet over medium-high heat for about 30 seconds.
3. Add the kale together with red pepper flakes to the skillet and cook for 2 minutes or until wilted.
4. Crack the eggs in a medium bowl, add salt and pepper and beat. Add the kale and thyme and mix well.
5. Transfer to 12 muffin tin, use the 2 tbsp. of oil and grease 8 muffin cups, sprinkle the tops with goat cheese.
6. Place in the oven and bake for 30 minutes or until set.

7. Serve warm. Keep the leftover in the fridge, use within a week and reheat before using.
Nutrition (per serving): 179 calories, | protein 10g, | carbohydrate 1.9g, | fiber 0.3g, sugar 0.3g, | fat 14g, | sodium 202.1mg | Potassium: 0mg |

Fluffy Lemon Ricotta Pancakes

Total time: 30 minutes
Prep time: 10 minutes
Cook time: 15 minutes
Servings: 4
Ingredients:
4 large eggs
1 cup whole-milk ricotta cheese
1 medium lemon
1/2 cup almond milk
1 tsp. baking powder
1 cup all-purpose flour
1 tbsp. granulated sugar
1/4 tsp. Sea salt
Unsalted butter, for cooking
For topping: fresh berries, citrus segments, maple syrup or lemon curd
Instructions:
1. Crack the eggs and separate the white egg from the yolks. Place the white egg in a medium and the egg yolks in another medium bowl.
2. Grate zest of 1 medium lemon and add to the egg yolk bowl. Add 3 tbsp. of lemon juice, almond milk and whole-milk ricotta cheese to the bowl and whisk well.
3. Add flour, baking powder, sugar and to the bowl and whisk until well mixed.
4. Beat the egg white with electric whisk for 3 minutes or until sturdy whisk.
5. Add 1/3 of the white egg to the egg yolk batter and stir with a rubber spatula and then gradually add in the rest of the egg white and stir until well combined.
6. Heat a nonstick skillet over medium heat and add the butter let it swirl to coat the bottom of the skillet.
7. Divide the batter into 4 portions and gently spread out each portion into rough 4 inches rounds, place in the pan at a time and cook for 3 minute on one side flip and cook for another 3 minutes.
8. Remove from heat and place in a plate and then repeat the process with the remaining batter.
9. Serve with any topping of choice. Enjoy!

Smashed Egg Toasts with Herby Lemon Yogurt

Total time: 20 minutes
Prep time: 5 minutes
Cook time: 15 minutes
Servings: 4

Ingredients:
1 clove garlic, Minced
1 medium lemon, finely grated and juiced
2 tbsp. finely chopped fresh chives, plus more for garnish
2 1/2 tbsp. finely chopped fresh basil leaves
8 large eggs
2 1/2 tbsp. finely chopped fresh dill
2 cups plain Greek yogurt
2 1/2 tbsp. extra-virgin olive oil
4 large slices sourdough bread (about 1-inch thick)
4 tbsp. unsalted butter, divided
3/4 tsp. kosher salt
1/2 tsp. freshly ground black pepper

Instructions:
1. Pour 5 liters of water in a pot and bring to a boil over medium-high heat.
2. Reduce the heat to low heat and let the water simmer for a while, gradually add all the eggs to the pot at once and let it cook for 6 minutes.
3. While the eggs are cooking, pour cold water on a bowl and add ice cubes to it.
4. Transfer the cooked eggs from the pot to the bowl of cold water with slotted spoon and let it sit for about 2 minutes and then peel the eggs under running water and put aside
5. Combine the basil, garlic, lemon juice, lemon zest, Greek yogurt, oil, fresh dill, chives, salt and pepper to a medium bowl and stir well.
6. Melt the butter in a large skillet over medium heat, add the slice bread and cook for 2 minutes on each side.
7. Remove from heat and place in a plate. Repeat the process with remaining butter and bread.
8. Spread the bread with yogurt mixture, top 2 eggs on each bread toast and use the back of a spoon to smash the eggs gently.
9. Sprinkle mixture with more herbs, oil, salt and black pepper. Enjoy!
Note: Store the leftover yogurt in an airtight container and keep in the fridge for 3 days.

Nutrition (per serving): 437 calories, | protein 23.5g, | carbohydrate 7.4g, | fiber 0.6g, sugar 5.5g, | fat 35.5g, | sodium 564.4mg | Potassium: 0mg |

Crispy White Beans with Greens and Poached Egg

Total time: 25 minute
Prep time: 10 minutes
Cook time: 15 minutes
Servings: 4

Ingredients:

3 tbsp. extra virgin olive oil, divided
4 large eggs, poached
1 cans cannellini beans, drained and rinsed
2 tsp. s za'atar, divided
1 medium bunch Swiss chard, stems removed and leaves thinly sliced
2 cloves garlic, minced
1/4 tsp. red pepper flakes, plus more for serving
1 tbsp. freshly squeezed lemon juice
1 tsp. kosher salt, divided

Instructions:

1. Heat 2 tbsp. of oil in a large skillet over medium-high heat for 1 minute.
2. Add the beans to the skillet, spread on even layer and cook for 4 minutes or until beans are browned on the bottom.
3. Add 1 tsp. of za'atar and 1/2 tsp. salt to the skillet and stir well. Spread out the beans again and continue cooking for 5 minutes, stir as needed.
4. Add the remaining 1 tbsp. of oil to the skillet. Add the chard, 1 tsp. of za'atar, garlic, red pepper flakes and 1/2 tsp. of salt. Cook and stir occasionally for 5 minutes or until chard is welded.
5. Remove the skillet from the heat and add the lemon juice and well to combine.
6. Divide the greens and beans among 4 serving bowls and top each portion with a poached egg, add more red pepper flakes and serve immediately. Enjoy!

Note: Store the left over in an air tight container and keep in the fridge. Make sure you use within 4 days.

Nutrition (per serving): 301 calories, | protein 15.5g, | carbohydrate 26.5g, | fiber 6.4g, sugar 1.5g, | fat 15.5g, | sodium 569.6mg | Potassium: 0mg |

Grain and mixed berries Salad

Total time: 65 minute
Prep time: 10 minutes
Cook time: 30 minutes
Servings: 8

Ingredients:
1 cup steel-cut oats
1/2 cup dry millet
1 cup dry golden quinoa
3 tbsp. olive oil, divided
1 (1-inch) piece fresh ginger, peeled and cut into coins
1/2 cup maple syrup
2 cups mixed berries
2 large lemons, zest and juice
2 cups hazelnuts, roughly chopped and toasted
1/4 tbsp. nutmeg
1 cup soy yogurt
Instructions:
1. Combine the quinoa, oats and millet in a fine strainer and rinse for 1 minute under running water and put aside.
2. Heat 1 tbsp. of oil in a medium saucepan over medium-high heat and the grains to the saucepan and cook for 3 minutes.
3. Pour 4 1/2 cups of clean water to the pan, add salt ginger coins, zest of lemon and 3/4 tsp. of salt to the pan and stir well.
4. Cover the pan and let it boil over medium heat for 2 minutes.
5. Reduce heat to low heat and let it simmer for 20 minutes. Remove from heat and let it sit for 5 minutes.
6. Take away the lid and fluff a fork. Remove the ginger and spread the grains on a large baking dish and let it cool for 30 minutes.
7. Transfer the cooled grains into a large bowl and add the lemon zest to the bowl and stir well.
8. Combine the 2 tbsp. of oil, lemon juice to a medium bowl and whisk until well mixed. Add the yogurt, nutmeg and maple syrup to the bowl and whisk well.
9. Pour mixture into the grains and stir until well coated. Add the mixed berries and toasted hazelnuts. Taste and make necessary adjustment.
10 Serve immediately or put in the fridge overnight so that the flavor will come out well. Enjoy.
Nutrition (per serving): 353 calories, | protein 9.6g, | carbohydrate 38g, | fiber 5.5g, sugar 12.6g, | fat 15.5g, | sodium 14.8mg | Potassium: 0mg |

Eggs with Summer Tomatoes, Zucchini, and Bell Peppers

Total time: 46 minute
Prep time: 10 minutes
Cook time: 36 minutes
Servings: 2

Ingredients:
1 tbsp. extra virgin olive oil
1 small yellow onion, halved and thinly sliced
1 clove garlic, minced
4 cups summer zucchini
2 large eggs
1 tsp. ground Spanish piquillo pepper
3 cups tomatoes, chopped
1 medium red bell pepper
Sea Salt to taste
Freshly ground black pepper
Instructions:
1. Heat the oil in a large heavy skillet over medium-high heat, add onion, stir and cook for 5 minutes or until is translucent, add the garlic and cook for 1 minute.
2. Add the squash and cook for 10 minutes or until soften and brown. Add the thyme, piquillo to the skillet and reduce the heat to low heat and let it simmer for about 20 minutes.
3. Remove the core and seed in the red bell pepper and cut into 1 inch pieces. Remove the skillet from the heat, sprinkle pepper with salt to taste and roast for 3 minutes.
4. Remove from heat and let it cool before serving. Crack the in a small bowl, add salt and pepper, heat oil in a skillet over medium heat, add the eggs and cook for about 2 minutes.
5. To serve, Divide veggies among 2 serving plates, top each plate egg and serve with buttered toast.
Note: You can use 3/4 cup of jarred roasted red peppers, if you did not prepare your own pepper, chop them into 1 inch pieces.
Nutrition (per serving): 226 calories, | protein 11.1g, | carbohydrate 20.6g, | fiber 6.3g, sugar 11.9g, | fat 12.5g, | sodium 1103mg | Potassium: 0mg |

Avocado and Egg Breakfast Pizza

Total time: 65 minute
Prep time: 10 minutes
Cook time: 30 minutes
Servings: 4
Ingredients:
1 tbsp. finely chopped cilantro
4 large eggs
1 1/2 tsp. lime juice
1 large Hass avocado, Halved, remove pit and cut in lengthwise
1/2 pound pizza dough, homemade

1 tbsp. extra virgin olive oil
1/8 tsp. salt
Instructions:
1. Scoop the flash of the avocado into a medium bowl and add lime juice, cilantro and salt and then mash with a fork until almost smooth but with a few chunks of avocados. Set aside.
2. Divide the homemade pizza dough into 4 equal parts. Place each part on a floured chopping board and roll into thin 6 inches circle.
3. Heat a seasoned cast iron skillet over medium-high heat until hot and place one of the circle pizza dough in the center of the heated skillet and cook until sides are browned and top surface is bubbly , about for 2 minutes turn and cook for another 2 minutes again. Remove from heat and transfer to a plate to cool off and then repeat the process with remaining dough.
4. Spread 1/4 avocado mixture on each cooked circle piece.
5. Crack the eggs in a medium bowl, add salt and heat oil a saucepan over medium heat, add the egg to the pan and cook for 2 minutes or as desires. Remove from heat and top each pizza with the egg. Serve right away. Enjoy!
Nutrition (per serving): 337 calories, | protein 12.3g, | carbohydrate 33.2g, | fiber 4.9g, sugar 1g, | fat 17.6g, | sodium 422.5mg | Potassium: 0mg |

Green Smoothie with Spinach, Almond Butter and Dates

Total time: 10 minute
Prep time: 10 minutes
Cook time: 0 minutes
Servings: 4
Ingredients:
1 banana, sliced and frozen (unfrozen is fine, too)
1 tbsp. almond butter
1 Medjool dates, pitted and torn into pieces,
 4 oz. spinach
1 cup unsweetened almond milk
Handful of ice
Pinch sea salt
1 tbsp. chia seeds, optional
1 tbsp. hemp seeds, optional
Instructions:
1. Combine all the ingredients in a bowl of a blender or food processor and blend until smooth, if too thick, add water or more almond milk to thin and blend again until your desired consistency is reached.

2. Transfer to a serving glass cup and enjoy immediately.

Low Carb Green Smoothie Bowl

This low carb and sugar free green smooth is healthy and so yummy
Total time: 5 minute
Prep time: 5 minutes
Cook time: 0 minutes
Servings: 1
Ingredients:
1 cup Spinach
1/2 scoop Collagen
1/2 tbsp. extra virgin olive oil
2 tbsp. Lemon juice
1/2 medium Avocado
3/4 cup unsweetened almond milk
3 tbsp. Besti Monk Fruit Allulose Blend
1/4 cup Ice cubes
TOPPINGS
1 tsp Hemp seeds
1 tsp Coconut flakes
1/2 tsp Chia seeds
Mixed berries
Instructions:
1. Combine all the recipes in a bowl of blender or food processor and blend smooth
2. Transfer to a serving bowl and top with the toppings and enjoy.
Nutrition (per serving): 319 calories, | protein 10g, | carbohydrate 15g, | fiber 10g, sugar 2g, | fat 26g, | sodium 0mg | Potassium: 0mg |

Peanut Butter and Kale with Flax Seeds Smoothie

Total time: 6 minute
Prep time: 5 minutes
Cook time: 1 minute
Servings: 2
Ingredients:
2 cups almond milk
2 frozen bananas
2 handfuls of kale
3 tbsp. peanut butter
1 tsp. cinnamon
1 tbsp. ground flax seeds
Instructions:

1. Combine all the ingredients in a bowl of a blender and blend until smooth and creamy
2. Transfer to a serving glass cup and enjoy.

Kale-Ginger Detox Smoothie
Total time: 2 minute
Prep time: 5 minutes
Cook time: 1 minute
Servings: 1
Ingredients:
1/2 cup frozen blueberries
2 tsp. ginger peeled and finely grated
1 ripe banana peeled and frozen
2 cups kale leaves loosely packed
1 cup unsweetened almond milk
1/8 tsp. ground cinnamon
2 tsp. Raw honey
1 tbsp. chia seeds optional
Instructions:
1. Combine all the ingredients in a bowl of blender or food processor and blend until smooth and creamy, add more almond milk or water if too thick and blend again until your desired consistency is reached.
2. Transfer to a serving glass cup and enjoy.

4 ingredients Smoothie

This smoothie is perfect with for breakfast, it will keep you refreshed for almost the whole day.
Total time: 2 minute
Prep time: 5 minutes
Cook time: 5 minutes
Servings: 2
Ingredients:
 1 cup frozen banana
 1 cup frozen mango
1 packed cup baby spinach
1 cup ice omit if using frozen fruit
1 cup milk
Instructions:
1. Combine all the ingredients in a bowl of a blender and blend until smooth and creamy.
 2. Divide smoothie among 2 serving glass cup and enjoy.

Nutrition (per serving): 231 calories, | protein 6.3g, | carbohydrate 45g, | fiber 4.6g, sugar 36.4g, | fat 2.5g, | sodium 71mg | Potassium: 0mg |

Walnut Toffee Tart

Serve this walnut toffee tart in any festive period. It is so impressive to serve.
Total time: 30 minutes
Prep time: 10 minutes
Cook time: 20 minutes
Servings: 12
Ingredients:
2 cups all-purpose flour
2 large egg yolks, lightly beaten
3 tbsp. sugar
1/4 cup cold milk
3/4 cup cold butter
For filling:
11/2 cups heavy whipping cream
2 cups coarsely chopped walnuts
1/2 tsp. ground cinnamon
1-1/2 cups sugar
1/4 tsp. salt
Instructions:
1. Preheat the oven to 375F°
2. Combine flour and sugar in a large bowl, add butter and mix until mixture looks like coarse crumbs.
3. Combine the milk and egg yolks in small bowl, mix well and add to the flour and continue mixing until well mixed.
4. Lightly rub flour in your hand onto the bottom and 1inch up the sides of a 12 inches tart pan with a removable bottom.
5. Line unpricked crust with a double thickness of heavy-duty foil and fill each with the mixture.
6. Place the pan on a baking sheet and bake until lightly brown on the edges, for about 15 minutes.
7. While the tart is baking, combine the cinnamon, cream, sugar and salt in a saucepan and let it boil over medium-high heat, stir often.
8. Remove the pan from heat and stir in the walnuts. Take off the foil from crust and pour the cinnamon mixture into the crust and continue baking until for 24 minutes or until golden brown.
9. Remove to a wire rack to cool off before storing in the fridge
10. Serve ad enjoy!
Nutrition (per serving): 529 calories, | protein 7 , | carbohydrate 48g, | fiber 2g, sugar 30g, | fat 4.2g, | sodium 153mg | Potassium: 0mg |

Walnut Ginger Tube Cake

You will love this walnut ginger cake
Total time: 60 minutes
Prep time: 20 minutes
Cook time: 40 minutes
Servings: 16
Ingredients:
1 cup packed brown sugar
1 cup hot brewed coffee
1/4 cup sour cream
1 cup olive oil
1 cup light molasses
2 large eggs, room temperature
31/4 cups all-purpose flour
21/2 tsp. baking soda
5 tsp. ground ginger
1/4 cup chopped ginger
11/2 tsp. ground cinnamon
1 tsp. salt
1 cup chopped walnuts, toasted
For Glaze:
2 cups confectioners' sugar
3- 4 tbsp. lemon juice
2 tsp. grated lemon zest
1 tbsp. chopped ginger
Instructions:
1. Preheat the oven to 350F°
2. Properly grease and lightly flour a 10 inches fluted tube pan.
3. Combine the brown sugar, coffee, olive oil, molasses and sour cream in a large bowl and beat until smooth. Add the eggs and continue beating until well mixed
4. Combine the flour, baking soda, ground ginger, cinnamon and salt into another large bowl and whisk well.
5. Slowly add the wet mixture into the flour mixture, add walnuts and ginger.
6. Transfer mixture to the pan and bake for 40 minutes. Let it sit for 10minutesbefore removing to a wire rack to cool completely.
7. To make the glaze, combine the confectioners' sugar, lemon juice and lemon zest in a small bowl and mix well.
8. Drizzle the glaze over the cake, sprinkle with more ginger. Serve and enjoy!

Nutrition (per serving): 465 calories, | protein 4g, | carbohydrate 68g, | fiber 1g, sugar 45g, |fat 20g, | sodium 369mg |Potassium: 0mg |

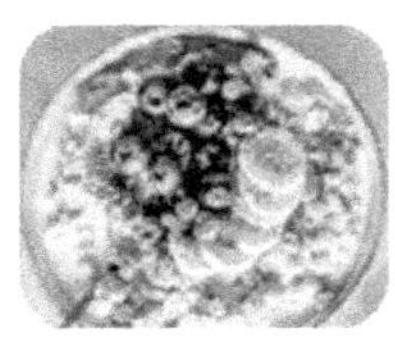

Sunflower Oatmeal

This recipe is so delicious! Your entire house hold will love it.
Total time: 52 minutes
Prep time: 20 minutes
Cook time: 12 minutes
Servings: 36
Ingredients:
1 cup white sugar
1 cup packed brown sugar
1/2 tsp. baking powder
1 cup butter, softened
2 cups all-purpose flour
2 large eggs
1 tsp. vanilla extract
1 tsp. baking soda
1 cup flaked coconut
2 cups rolled oats
1 cup roasted and salted sunflower seeds
Instructions:
1. Preheat the oven to 350°F.
2. Combine the white sugar, brown sugar and butter in medium bowl and whisk well until smooth and creamy.
3. Beat the eggs one after the other and add the vanilla and stir well.
4. Combine the dry ingredients, the flour, baking soda and baking powder in a bowl.
5. Combine the cream mixture and the dry mixture together and mix well until smooth.
6. Add the sunflower seeds, rolled oats and mix well and then add the coconut flakes.
7. Place 2 tbsp. of the dough into a cookie sheets, don't over filled the cookie sheets, repeat until no more dough.
8. Place the cookie sheets into the heated oven and bake for 12 minutes or until edges are brown.

9. Let the cookies set for 2 minutes before removing to a wire racks to cool down completely. Serve.

Nutrition (per serving): 166.7 calories, | protein 2.5g, | carbohydrate 21.9g, | fiber 1g, sugar 0g, | fat 6g, | sodium 0mg | Potassium: 0mg |

SOUP RECIPES

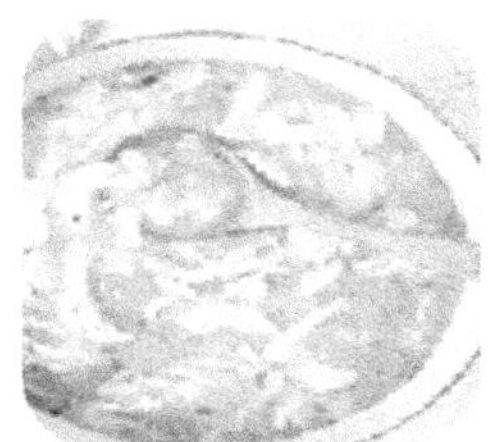

Pumpkin, apple and shallot Soup

This pumpkin and shallot recipe is yummy and quick to prepare.

Total time 45 minutes
Prep time: 10 minutes
Cook time: 35 minutes
Servings: 6

Ingredients:

1 sugar pumpkin (cut in half and scrape out the seed and fibers with spoon)
2 shallots (peel, root removed and cut in half)
2 large Granny Smith apples (cut in half and core)
1 tsp. granulated sugar
1/4 tsp. freshly grated nutmeg
3 tbsp. extra virgin olive oil
4 cups chicken broth (or vegetable broth, hot)
1/2 cup heavy whipping cream
1/8 tsp. ground cayenne pepper
1 tsp. sea salt
1 tsp. freshly ground black pepper

For garnish

Toasted pepitas
1/3 cup sour cream

Instructions:

1. Preheat the oven to 400°F. Line a large rimmed baking dish with aluminum foil and position the baking dish in the middle of the oven rack.

2. Properly brush the pumpkin halves with oil and season with salt and pepper. Brush the cut side of shallot and apple with oil.
3. Place the pumpkin in the prepared baking dish, let the cut side down. Place the shallots and apple beside the pumpkin and let the cut side down.
4. Roast for 30 minutes or until pumpkin is softened
5. Remove from oven and transfer to a bowl of blender or food processor and process until smooth.
6. Return back to the heat and add the cream, nutmeg, sugar, cayenne pepper and broth and let it heat through. Taste and season with salt and pepper as needed.
7. To serve, garnish with Toasted pepitas and sour cream and enjoy!
Nutrition (per serving): 280 calories, | protein 6g, | carbohydrate 30g, | fiber 3g, sugar 0g, | fat 18g, | sodium 470mg | Potassium: 0mg |

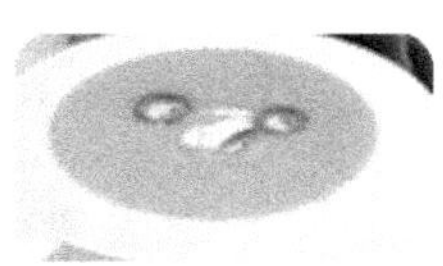

Crockpot Lentil Soup

This lentil soup is very easy to make. It's made with carrots, onions, squash, garlic, olive oil, and lentils, so simple and clean soup.

Total time: 6 hours
Prep time: 30 minutes
Cook time: 5 hours 30 minutes
Servings: 8
Ingredients:
For the Crockpot:
2 cups butternut squash peeled and cubed
2 cups carrots peeled and sliced
1 cup green lentils
2 cups potatoes, finely chopped
2 cups celery, finely chopped
3/4 cup yellow split peas
1 onion finely chopped
2 tsp. herbs de provence
5 cloves garlic minced
8–10 cups chicken broth
1 tsp. salt
2–3 cups kale (removes steam and thinly chopped)
1 cup parsley (finely chopped)
1/2 cup olive oil
1tbsp lemon juice

Instructions:
1. Combine all the ingredients in a Crockpot, and close the lid and cook for 6 hours on high heat or 8 hours on low heat.
2. In a high power blender, place 4 cups of the soup, add olive oil and blend until roughly smooth.
3. Return the soup back to the pot and stir well. Add the parsley, kale and stir well.
4. Remove from heat and let cool to room temperature.
5. Top with vinegar, sherry and lemon juice and then serve with crusty wheat bread. Enjoy!
Nutrition (per serving): 322 calories, | protein 10.8g, |carbohydrate 39.5g, | fiber 13.2g, sugar 0g, |fat 14g, | sodium 0mg |Potassium: 0mg |

Turmeric Chicken Soup

This recipe is easy and fast to make, delicious soup to enjoy with your family and friends.
Total time: 55 minutes
Prep time: 20 minutes
Cook time: 35 hours 30 minutes
Servings: 12
Ingredients:
1 1/2 pounds chicken breast, boneless and skinless
3 cups broccoli florets
2 quarts chicken broth
1/4 cup chopped parsley
2 1/2 cups sliced carrots
1/4 teaspoon ground turmeric
1 large onion, finely chopped
2 tbsp. olive oil
2 cups chopped celery
1/4 - 1/2 tsp. crushed red pepper
1 1/2 cups frozen peas
3 tbsp. fresh ginger, shredded or grated
4 garlic cloves minced
1 tbsp. apple cider vinegar
Sea saltto taste
Freshly ground pepper to taste
Instructions:
1. Heat the oil in a saucepan over medium heat; add onions, ginger, celery, and garlic and cook until soften, for 6 minutes
2. Add the chicken, apple cider vinegar, carrots, turmeric, crushed red pepper, broth and salt to taste.

3. Lower the heat to low and let it simmer until the chicken is cooked through, about for 20-22 minutes.
4. Carefully remove the chicken with tongs to a chopping board to cool down.
5. Add the broccoli, parsley and peas to the pot and let it simmer for 8 minutes until broccoli is softened.
6. Shred or slice the chicken and return back to the pot soup and let it simmer for more 12 minutes, until the broccoli is softened, Season with salt and pepper to taste.
7. Scoop to a serving plate and serve immediately. Enjoy!
Nutrition (per serving): 91 calories, | protein 9g, | carbohydrate 65g, | fiber 1g, sugar 0g, |fat 2g, | sodium 0mg | Potassium: 0mg |

Broccoli Detox Soup

This soup is packed with lot of fiber, minerals and vitamins. So delicious!!
Total time: 15 minutes
Prep time: 5 minutes
Cook time: 10 minutes
Servings: 2
Ingredients:
2 cups broccoli florets
2 garlic cloves crushed
2 celery stalks, diced
1 onion, diced
1 cup greens spinach, kale, beet greens or any other available
1 parsnip washed, peeled and thinly chopped
1 carrot washed, peeled and thinly chopped
1/2 lemon
1 tbsp. chia seeds
1 tsp. coconut oil
2 cups drinkable water
1/2 tsp. sea salt
For garnishing
Toasted mixed seeds and nuts
1 tsp. coconut milk
Instructions:
1. Heat coconut oil in a large soup pot over medium heat; add onion, garlic, celery sticks, carrot, broccoli and parsnip to the pot.
2. Reduce the heat to low heat and let it simmer for 5 minutes, stir often.
3. Add the water, let it boil and then close the pot with a lid and let is simmer until veggies are tender, for about 7 minutes.

4. Add the greens and stir well. Remove from heat and transfer to a blender, add the lemon juice and chia seed and then blend until very smooth and creamy.

1. Garnish with toasted seeds, top with coconut milk and serve immediately.

Nutrition (per serving): 182calories, | protein 5.5g, | carbohydrate 35g.1, | fiber 10g, sugar 2g, | fat 4.2g, | sodium 456mg | Potassium: 408mg |

Broccoli Cheese Soup

This broccoli cheese recipe is so comforting, creamy and simple to make. Yummy! You will love it.

Total time: 30 minutes

Prep time: 10 minutes

Cook time: 20 minutes

Servings: 6

Ingredients:

5 cup broccoli florets cut into 1/2-inch florets and finely chop the stem

1/2 onion, thinly chopped.

2 large carrots, thinly chopped.

1/4 cup all-purpose flour

2 cloves garlic, minced

2 stalks celery, thinly chopped.

2 cups whole milk

2 tbsp. salted butter

1 tsp. Dijon mustard

2 1/2 cups chicken broth

3/4tsp. sea salt

1/2 tsp. freshly ground black pepper

2 cups shredded cheddar cheese minced, (for serving)

Instructions:

1. Melt the butter in a Dutch oven over medium high-heat and add onion, celery, carrots, and salt and cook for 7 minutes or until veggies are softened.

2. Add the mustard and garlic and continues cook and stir for about a minute or until fragrant

3. Add the flour to the pot and stir until well coated.

4. Add the milk and broth to the pot and stir until flour is dissolved, add salt and pepper followed by the broccoli and bring to a boil, stir occasionally.

5. Reduce heat to low heat, cover pot and let it simmer for about 10 minutes or until broccoli is soften, stir once or 2 times.

6. Put off the heat but let the pot still be on the burner. Add 1/2 of the cheese, stir and let it melt before adding the remaining and stir until completely melted.

7. To serve, spoon soup to a serving plate, sprinkle with parsley, freshly ground pepper and salt if you want. Enjoy!

Nutrition (per serving): 310 calories, | protein 17g, | carbohydrate 17g, | fiber 3g, sugar 0g, | fat 20g, | sodium 890mg | Potassium: 0mg |

Creamy Cauliflower Soup

Total time: 39 minutes
Prep time: 15 minutes
Cook time: 24 minutes
Servings: 6

Ingredients:
1 medium white onion (diced)
3 garlic cloves (peeled and minced)
1 large carrot (1/2" quarter chop)
2 celery stalks (1/2" chop)
1/4 cup extra virgin olive oil
3 Ib. cauliflowers (broken into florets)
5 cups vegetable broth
1/2tsp. lemon zest
1/2 cup heavy cream
1/8 tsp. Nut Meg
1/4 cup fresh Italian parsley (packed, minced)
1 tsp. sea salt
1 tsp. freshly ground pepper

Instructions:
1. Heat oil in Dutch oven over medium-high heat. Add the onions, garlic, celery and carrots to the pot cook and stir constantly for 4 minutes or until onions are translucent.

2. Add the Cauliflower and vegetable broth to the pot and stir until well mixed.

3. Lower the heat to medium heat, cover the pot and let it simmer until cauliflowers soften for about 20 minutes.

4. Put off the heat and then add cream, nutmeg, lemon zest and salt to the pot.

5. Transfer to a blender and blend until creamy and let some cauliflower florets remain in the soup.

6. Return the soup back to the pot and add the parsley and serve immediately.

Nutrition (per serving): 270 calories, | protein 10g, |carbohydrate 17g, | fiber 6g, sugar 0g, |fat 19g, | sodium 114mg | Potassium: 0mg |

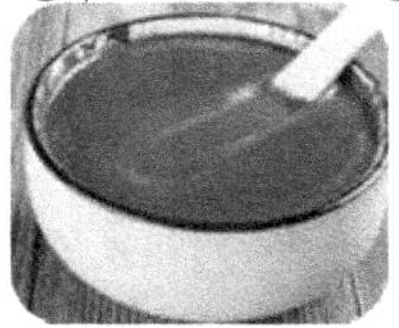

Quick Black Sesame Soup

Total time: 15 minutes
Prep time: 15 minutes
Cook time: 0 minutes
Servings: 4
Ingredients:
1/2 cup toasted black sesame seeds (plus more to serve)
2 cups drinkable water
1/2 cup unsalted cashews
2 tbsp. rolled oats
2 tbsp. Chinese rock sugar
Instructions:
1. In a bowl of a power blender, combine the water, cashews, sesame seeds, oats, and sugar.
2. Cover the blender with a lid and blend until blender turn off by itself or for 4 minutes, starting from the lowest speed and increase to the highest.
3. The soup will be hot from the blender. Transfer to a serving plate, let sit for a few minutes and then top with crushed nuts, toasted sesame seeds, shredded coconut. Enjoy!
Nutrition (per serving): 200 calories, | protein 6 g, |carbohydrate 12g, | fiber 3g, sugar 0g, |fat 16g, | sodium 15mg | Potassium: 0mg |

Healthy Silky Tortilla

Total time: 35 minutes
Prep time: 15 minutes
Cook time: 20 minutes
Servings: 5
Ingredients:
3 tbsp. extra virgin olive oil, divided
3 cloves garlic
1 cup white onion, finely chopped
1 jalapeno pepper Remove seed and finely chopped
1/2 tsp. red pepper flakes
12 oz. salsa

1 1/2 cups vegetable broth
14.5 oz. fire roasted tomatoes
1/2 cup black beans
1 Ib. chicken breast, cooked and shredded
Jalapeno peppers sliced fresh
3 corn tortillas cut into thin strips
Shredded cheddar cheese
Instructions:
1. Heat 1 tbsp. of oil in a skillet, add onions, garlic, Jalapeno and red pepper to the skillet and cook for 4 minutes.
2. Transfer to a blender and add the vegetable broth, salsa, roasted, black beans and tomatoes and pulse on speed until puree, for about 6 times.
3. Return to a pot and simmer on a medium heat for 15 minutes.
4. In a heavy skillet, heat the 2 tbsp. of oil, add the tortilla chips and fry until crisp. Drain chips on a paper tower until ready to use.
5. Divide soup among 5 serving plate and top with tortilla strips, shredded chicken, cheese and fresh pepper. Enjoy!
Nutrition (per serving): 350 calories, | protein 33g, | carbohydrate 25g, | fiber 7g, sugar 0g, |fat 14g, | sodium 1000mg | Potassium: 0mg |
Sodium| Potassium: 0mg

Hearty Lentil

With a few ingredients you will put together this hearty lentil soup and it will keep you warmth in a winter time. You can make it ahead and take it any time of the day. You can also modify this recipe according to your taste.
Total time: 60 minutes
Prep time: 20 minutes
Cook time: 40 minutes
Servings: 12
Ingredients:
1 Ib. lentils
1 Ib. bacon, sliced
1 cup celery chopped, with leaves
1 cup carrots, chopped
2 cloves garlic, minced
2large tomatoes, washed and diced
3 quarts water
1 1/2 tsp. Sea salt
For the optional ingredients
Bay leaf, Basil, Lemon juice, hot sauce
Instructions:

1. In a skillet over medium heat, add the bacon and garlic and cook until bacon is tender.
2. Remove bacon from heat, drain fat, return skillet to the heat and then add the rest of the ingredients and let it boil over medium-high heat.
3. Lower the heat and let it simmer until lentils are softened but firm, for about 30 minutes.
4. Transfer half of the mixture to a blender and puree until creamy and then return back to the pot.
5. Serve with optional ingredients if you want. Enjoy!
Nutrition (per serving): 320 calories, | protein 29g, | carbohydrate g, 29 | fiber 12g, sugar 0g, | fat 17g, | sodium 660mg | Potassium: 0mg |

Healthy Carrot Ginger Soup

This carrot ginger soup will keep you warmth for the day.
Total time: 35 minutes
Prep time: 20 minutes
Cook time: 40 minutes
Servings: 4
Ingredients:
6 cups carrots, peeled and cubed
2 tbsp. extra-virgin olive oil
2 cups diced yellow onion
5 cups vegetable broth
2 tsp. minced garlic
2 tbsp. minced fresh ginger
3/4 cup full-fat canned almond milk
1 tsp. sea salt
Instructions:
1. Heat oil in a large saucepan over medium-high heat and add onion, garlic, 1/4 tsp. of salt and cook until onion is softened and translucent, for about 5 minutes.
2. Add ginger and carrot to the saucepan and cook until equally coated and fragrant, for 1 minute.
3. Add the broth and rest of the salt and let it boil over high heat
4. Lower the heat to medium heat, partially cover the saucepan and let it simmer until carrot is softened, for about 20 minutes.
5. Remove from heat and add 1/2 cup of almond milk and let it slightly cool down.
6. Transfer to a blender and blend on high until smooth and creamy, for about 1 minute (you can blend in batches)
7. Return to the saucepan, taste and adjust season and then warm on low heat.

8. Spoon soup in a serving plate and add remaining of almond milk and swirl it with a butter knife. Enjoy!

Nutrition (per serving): 220 calories, | protein 10g, | carbohydrate 27g, | fiber 6g, sugar 0g, | fat 16g, | sodium 543mg | Potassium: 0mg |

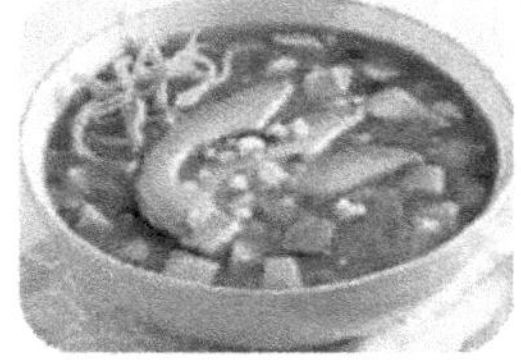

Chicken Tortilla avocado Soup

Total time: 20 minutes
Prep time: 10 minutes
Cook time: 10 minutes
Servings: 5

Ingredients:
2 cloves garlic, finely chopped
1 tbsp. extra virgin olive oil
1 corn tortilla, 7" in length, torn into pieces
1 medium yellow onion, finely chopped
15 oz. diced fire roasted tomatoes with juice
4 oz. diced mild green chilies
2 cups chicken stock
2 tsp. chili powder
1 tsp. ground cumin
1 lime (juiced and peel grated)
1/4 cup chopped fresh cilantro
1 cup tortilla chips
2 cups cooked chicken, chopped
1 avocado, halved, pitted, peeled and diced
1/2 cup shredded Monterey Jack cheese
Sea salt to taste

Instructions:
1. Heat the olive oil in a skillet over medium-high heat and add onion, garlic and little salt, cover the skillet and cook until soften, for about 8 minutes. Remove from heat and set aside to cool.
2. Combine the torn tortilla, chiles, tomatoes, stock, cumin, chili powder, lime peel, cilantro and juice, and 1 tsp. of salt to a bowl of the blender. Add the onion and garlic mixture to the blender, cover with lid.
3. Start from the lowest speed and slowly increase to highest, blend for 5 minutes or until mixture is smooth and rising steam is noticeable.

4. Add the tortilla chips and chicken to the blender bowl and pulse for 3 times.

5. Spoon to a serving plate, garnish with cheese and avocado slices then and serve immediately. Enjoy!

Note: to store, let the tortilla chips cool off completely, then transfer to an airtight container and store in the fridge. Make sure you within a week. You can also freeze for up to 3 month. Add tortilla chips when warming.

Nutrition (per serving): 370 calories, | protein 24g, | carbohydrate 27g, | fiber 6g, sugar 0g, | fat 22g, | sodium 440mg | Potassium: 0mg |

Mixed Veggies Soup

This recipe is healthy and perfect for either lunch or dinner. It's yummy and the best way to enjoy your vegetable. Very easy to prepare

Total time: 55 minutes

Prep time: 15 minutes

Cook time: 40 minutes

Servings: 6

Ingredients:

2 carrots, diced

1/2 cup yellow onion, diced

1 tbsp. extra virgin olive oil

2 small zucchini, diced

2 celery stalks, diced

2 cloves garlic, minced

3 1/2 cup crushed tomatoes

4 cups vegetable broth

1 1/2 cup cannellini beans, drained and rinsed

1 tsp. dried oregano

1/2 cup small shell pasta

1 cup fresh baby spinach stems removed and thinly chopped

Instructions:

1. In a saucepan over medium low-heat, heat oil. Add the onion, garlic, celery, carrots, zucchini to the saucepan and cook for 5 minutes or until veggies start to soften.

2. Add the vegetable broth and tomatoes to the saucepan and let it boil over high heat.

3. Lower the heat to low heat and add the oregano and beans and let simmer uncovered for about 20 minutes.

4. Add the shell pasta to the saucepan and cook for more 8 minutes. Add the baby spinach, stir and cook until spinach is wilts, for 1 minute.

5. Remove from heat and serve.

Nutrition (per serving): 190 calories, | protein 3g, | carbohydrate 34g, | fiber 5g, sugar 0g, | fat 22g, | sodium 820mg | Potassium: 0mg |

Carrot and Cabbage Soup

This recipe is easy to make and packed with flavor.

Total time: 41 minutes

Prep time: 15 minutes

Cook time: 31 minutes

Servings: 6

Ingredients:

2 tbsp. extra-virgin olive oil

1 cup chopped carrots

1 cup of sliced fennel, reserve the fronds for garnish

1/2 cup chopped onion

2 tsp. minced garlic

1/2 tsp. ground coriander

1/2 tsp.sea salt

6 cups vegetable broth

1 tsp. basil,

1 can diced tomatoes

1 tsp. dried oregano

1 can unsalted cannellini beans, rinsed

2 cloves garlic, minced

1 1/2 Ib. cabbage, chopped

2 tsp. sugar

1 tsp. chopped fresh oregano

Lemon zest for garnish

Instructions:

1. In a large heavy pot over medium-high heat, heat the oil and add the onion, carrot and fennel to the pot, cook and stir, once or twice for 5 minutes or until veggies are soften.

2. Add the garlic and season with salt, stir and cook for 1 minute more or until aromatic heat

3. Add tomatoes and vegetable broth. Let it boil over medium heat. Add the cabbage.

4. Reduce heat to low heat and cook, stirring occasionally, for about 25 minutes.

5. Add sugar, oregano and bean to the pot and cook for about 3 minutes. Add the remaining fennel fronds and lemon zest and serve right away. Enjoy!

Nutrition (per serving): 205 calories, | protein 6.2g, | carbohydrate 31g, | fiber 9.6g, sugar 14.5g, | fat 22g, | sodium 425mg | Potassium: 669.8mg |

Spicy Chicken and Kale

Total time: 45 minutes
Prep time: 15 minutes
Cook time: 30 minutes
Servings: 5
Ingredients:
2 tbsp. extra virgin olive oil
1 red onion (peeled and chopped)
1 fennel bulb (cored and sliced)
3 cloves garlic (minced)
1 1/2 Ib. chicken breast, cut into bite size pieces
3 1/2cups diced tomatoes
4 cups chicken broth
1 cup dry white wine
4 cups kale (chopped)
1/4 tsp. crushed red pepper
6 oz. plain Greek yogurt
1 1/2 tbsp. extra virgin olive oil
1 cup basil leaves
Sea Salt to taste
Freshly ground black pepper
Instructions:
1. Heat oil in large pot over medium-high heat add onions, and fennel to the pot and cook for 4 minutes, add garlic and cook until the veggies are soften, for about more 3 minutes
2. Remove the veggies or push it aside and add the chicken and cook until almost cooked, for 5 minutes.
3. Add the chicken broth, tomatoes together with the juice, kale, wine, red pepper, Salt and pepper to taste. Bring to boil over medium-high heat, reduce heat to medium-low and let it simmer for 20 minutes.
4. While the soup is simmering, Combine the oil, yogurt and basil leave to a blender bowl, add a pinch of salt and blend until smooth.
5. To serve, spoon soup in a serving plate with yogurt and basil mixture on top and enjoy!

Nutrition (per serving): 400 calories, | protein 37g, | carbohydrate 22g, | fiber 5g, sugar 0g, | fat 17g, | sodium 430mg | Potassium: 0mg |

Lentil Soup with Kale

This recipe is hearty, healthy and packed with nutrients
Total time: 45 minutes
Prep time: 15 minutes
Cook time: 30 minutes
Servings: 4
Ingredients:
1 cup red lentils
2 tomatoes finely chopped
1 1/4 cups chopped kale leaves firmly packed
4 big garlic cloves finely chopped
1 onion finely chopped
1/2 tsp. cumin powder
2/4 tsp. red chili powder
1/2 teaspoon ground sumac
1/4 +1/8 tsp. turmeric powder
1/8tsp. ground cinnamon
1/2 tbsp. extra virgin olive oil
2 tbsp. parsley leaves chopped
4-5 cups water
Cilantro chopped to garnish
Sea salt to taste
Instructions:
1. Heat oil in a saucepan over medium-high heat and add the onion and garlic to the saucepan and cook for 2 minutes.
2. Add the tomatoes and cook for more 2 minutes. Add the kale and cook for 2 minutes. Add lentils and mix well.
3. Add the red chili powder, cumin powder, cinnamon powder, turmeric powder and ground sumac to the pan and season with salt as needed, mix well and cook for 1 minute.
4. Add the parsley leaves and water cover the pan with a lid and cook for about 25 minutes over medium heat or until lentil is done cooking. Put off the heat and let it cool down slightly.
5. Transfer half of the soup to a blender when it is a bit cooled and blend until smooth paste.
6. Return the blended soup back to the pan and mix well.
7. Reduce the heat to low heat and let it simmer for 10 minutes. Remove from heat and spoon into a serving plate, garnish with cilantro and serve warm with some pita bread on side. Enjoy!
Nutrition (per serving): 233 calories, | protein 13g, | carbohydrate 32g, | fiber 14g, sugar 2g, | fat 17g, | sodium 28mg | Potassium: 595mg |

Broccoli Cheese Soup

This broccoli cheese is perfect and keeps you warm all the day.
Total time: 40 minutes
Prep time: 10 minutes
Cook time: 30 minutes
Servings: 4
Ingredients:
1 large bunch broccoli, cut into florets
1 tablespoon extra olive oil
2 cloves garlic, finely chopped
3 cups vegetable broth
1 teaspoon fresh thyme leaves, finely chopped
1 medium onion, finely diced
1/2 teaspoon turmeric powder
1 cup sharp cheddar, shredded
1 cup heavy cream
Stale bread, cut into small dices (to make the croutons)
Salt and pepper to taste
Instructions:
1. In a large pot over medium-high heat, heat the oil when is heated add the broccoli and sauté for about 5 minutes or until lightly brown.
2. Add the onion, garlic, and sauté for more 2 minutes.
3. Add the thyme, turmeric powder broth to the pot and bring to boil.
4. Cover the pot and lower the heat and let it simmer for about 15 minutes
5. Preheat the oven to 400°F, place 1 tbsp. of oil in a baking dish and toast in the oven for about 8 minutes.
6. Place the bacon in a skillet and fry. When is done frying drain out the fat and cut the bacon into small bits. Put the bacon and croutons aside.
7. Add the cheese and cream to the soup pot and mix well. Taste and add salt and pepper to taste.
8. Transfer to a blender or food processor and blend until smooth.
9. Transfer to a serving plate and garnish with croutons and bacon. Enjoy!

SMOOTIES RECIPES

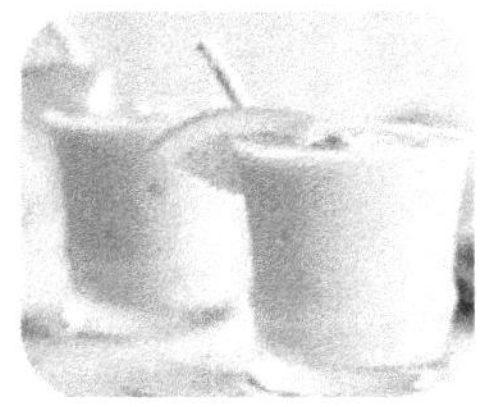

Green yogurt and Kale Smoothie

This recipe is loaded with protein; the Greek yogurt will boost your healthy
Total time: 10 minutes
Prep time: 5 minutes
Cook time: 0 minutes
Servings: 4
Ingredients:
1 cup chopped kale
1/2 unsweetened almond milk
11/2 cup frozen pineapple chunks
1/2 cup Green yogurt
1 tsp. honey
Instructions:
1. Combine the kale, almond milk, pineapple chunks, yogurt and honey in a blender bowl or food processor and until smooth and frothy.
2. Transfer to a serving glass cup and enjoy.
Nutrition (per serving): 296 calories, | protein 14g, |carbohydrate 45g, | fiber 5g, sugar 8,5g, |fat 4g, | sodium 0mg |Potassium: 0mg |

Pineapple and Grapefruit Smoothie

This smoothie is packed with nutrients and quick to prepare.
Total time: 10 minutes
Prep time: 5 minutes
Cook time: 0 minutes
Servings: 2
Ingredients:
1/2 cup frozen pineapple chunks
1/2 cup fat-free Greek yogurt
1/2 naval orange, segmented, plus more
1 tsp. vanilla extract
1/2 ruby grapefruit, segmented plus more
For garnishing
Coconut flakes,
Chopped cashews
Chia seed
Instructions:
1. Combine all the ingredients in a blender or food processor and process until smooth.
2. Divide mixture among 2 serving bowl and top each bowl with additional grapefruit and orange.

3. Garnish with coconut flakes, chia seed and chopped cashews. And enjoy.
Nutrition (per serving): 240calories, | protein 12g, |carbohydrate 31g, | fiber 5g, sugar 19g, |fat 8g, | sodium 10mg | Potassium: 0mg |

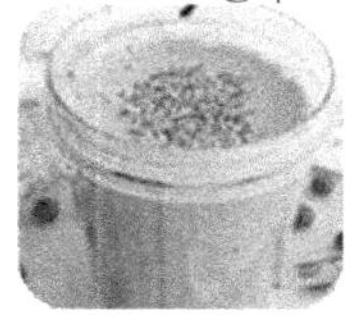

Kale and Blueberry Smoothie

This recipe is so refreshing
Total time: 10 minutes
Prep time: 5 minutes
Cook time: 0 minutes
Servings: 3
Ingredients:
4 slices fresh or frozen peaches
1 cup chilled almond
1/4 cup blueberries,
Handful of kale
1/4 tsp. ground cinnamon
Instructions:
1. Combine all the ingredients in a bowl of a blender or food processor and blend until smooth.
2. Transfer to serving plate and serve.
Nutrition (per serving): 170 calories, | protein 8.5g, |carbohydrate 26g, | fiber 4g, sugar 17g, |fat 4g, | sodium 10mg |Potassium: 0mg |

Blueberry-Soy and Banana- Smoothie

This smoothie is so healthy and loaded with flavor.
Total time: 10 minutes
Prep time: 5 minutes
Cook time: 0 minutes
Servings: 3
Ingredients:
1/2 cup frozen blueberries,
1 1/4 cups light soy milk
1/2 frozen banana,
1 tsp. pure vanilla extract
Instructions:
1. Combine all the ingredients all the bowl of a blender or food processor and blend until smooth,

2. Transfer to serving glass cup and enjoy!
Nutrition (per serving): 125 calories, | protein 3g, | carbohydrate 26g, | fiber 2g, sugar 11g, | fat 4g, | sodium 0mg | Potassium: 0mg |

Oatmeal and Peaches Smoothie

Total time: 10 minutes
Prep time: 5 minutes
Cook time: 0 minutes
Servings: 2
Ingredients:
1/2 cup Greek yogurt
1/2 cup almond milk
1/2 cup rolled oats
1/2 frozen banana
1 cup frozen peaches
1/2 cup ice cube
Instructions:
1. Combine all the ingredients in a bowl of blender or food processor and blend until smooth and creamy.
2. Transfer to a serving glass cup and serve.
Note: Save the left over in the fridge and try to use within a week
Nutrition (per serving): 217 calories, | protein 11g, | carbohydrate 33g, | fiber 4g, sugar 5.5g, | fat 4g, | sodium 0mg | Potassium: 0mg |

3 ingredients Smoothie

This pineapple smooth will surely satisfy your ice cream cone cravings, so yummy!
Total time: 10 minutes
Prep time: 5 minutes
Cook time: 0 minutes
Servings:4
Ingredients:
1 cup almond milk
1 cup pineapple chunks
6 ice cube
Instructions:
1. Combine the 3 ingredients in a bowl of a blender or mini food processor and pulse until smooth and creamy.
2. Transfer to a serving glass cup and serve, enjoy!
Note: Save the left over in the fridge and try to use within a week
Nutrition (per serving): 283 calories, 13g protein, 53.5g carbohydrates, 2g fiber, 48gg sugar, 3.5g fat, 4 g 0 mg sodium

Cucumber and grape Smoothie

This smoothie is quick and easy to prepare. Its makes a sip worthy snack
Total time: 10 minutes
Prep time: 5 minutes
Cook time: 0 minutes
Servings: 4
Ingredients:
1 medium English cucumber (peeled and sliced)
), 1 cup seedless green grapes
1 1/2 cups unsweetened almond milk
2 medium stalks celery (peeled and sliced)
1 Tbsp. honey
Instructions:
1. Combine all the ingredients in a bowl of a blender or mini food processor and until smooth and creamy.
2 transfer to a glass cup and enjoy
Note: Save the left over in the fridge and try to use within a week
Nutrition (per serving): 124 calories, | protein 2g, | carbohydrate 26g, | fiber 2g, sugar 21g, |fat 0g, | sodium 0mg | Potassium: 0mg |

Carrot and Apricots Smoothie

This smoothie recipe is loaded with vitamins and taste good. You will love it.
Total time: 10 minutes
Prep time: 5 minutes
Cook time: 0 minutes
Servings: 4
Ingredients:
1/4 cup grated carrot
2 chopped dried apricots
1/2 cup ice cubes
1/2 cup whole milk Greek yogurt
1 tsp. honey
1 fresh apricot (pitted and coarsely chopped)
1/2 tsp. cinnamon
Instructions:
1. Combine all the ingredients in the bowl of blender or food processor and blend until smooth and creamy
2. Transfer to a serving glass cup and enjoy.
Note: Save the left over in the fridge and try to use within a week
Nutrition (per serving): 130 calories, | protein 8g, | carbohydrate 21g, | fiber 3g, sugar 17g, |fat 0g, | sodium 0mg | Potassium: 0mg |

Kiwi and Banana Smoothie

This recipe help to replenish your energy and keep you rehydrated. You will like it
Total time: 10 minutes
Prep time: 5 minutes
Cook time: 0 minutes
Servings: 4
Ingredients:
1 kiwi (peeled and cut into pieces)
1 medium banana (Peeled and cut into pieces)
1 cup unsweetened almond milk
1 scoop vanilla whey protein powder
1/2 cup coconut water
1 cup spinach
Instructions:
1. Combine all the ingredients in a bowl of a blender or food processor and pulse until smooth and creamy.
2. Divide smoothie among 4 serving glass cup and enjoy immediately.
Nutrition (per serving): 304 calories, | protein 22g, | carbohydrate 47g, | fiber 7g, sugar 8g, | fat 0g, | sodium 0mg | Potassium: 0mg |

Strawberries and Oat Smoothie

This recipe is satisfying and it is quick and easy to prepare. It will keep you full for almost the whole day.
Total time: 10 minutes
Prep time: 5 minutes
Cook time: 0 minutes
Servings: 4
Ingredients:
1 banana, peeled and sliced
2 cups frozen strawberries
1/2 cup orange juice
1/2 cup rolled oats
1/2 cup orange juice
1 Tbsp. honey
Instructions:
1. Combine all the ingredients in a bowl of a blender food processor and blend until smooth and creamy.
2. Divide smoothie among 4 serving glass cups and serve right away.
Nutrition (per serving): 171 calories, | protein 5g, | carbohydrate 36g, | fiber 3.5g, sugar 23g, | fat 2g, | sodium 0mg | Potassium: 0mg |

Pineapple and banana Smoothie

This recipe perfect in calming your nerves and it is quick and easy smooth for keeping you satisfying for a long time.

Total time: 10 minutes
Prep time: 5 minutes
Cook time: 0 minutes
Servings: 1

Ingredients:

1/2 cup pineapple chunks
1/4 cup refrigerated sugar-free coconut milk
1/4 cup Greek yogurt
1/4 cup orange juice
1/4 large banana
4 ice cube

Instructions:

1. Combine all the ingredients in the bowl of a blender and or food processor and blend until mixture is smooth and creamy.
2. Transfer smoothie in a serving glass cup and serve immediately.

Nutrition (per serving): 156 calories, | protein 6g, | carbohydrate 29g, | fiber 2g, sugar 21g, | fat 3g, | sodium 0mg | Potassium: 0mg |

Healthy Green Ginger Smoothie

Total time: 10 minutes
Prep time: 5 minutes
Cook time: 0 minutes
Servings: 2

Ingredients:

1 chopped Granny Smith apple
2 cups packed baby spinach
2 Tbsp. hemp seeds
3/4 cup coconut water
1/4 cup lemon juice
3 tsp. minced ginger
1 1 1/2 cup ice cubes
Tsp. raw honey

Instructions:

1. Combine all the ingredients in the bowl of a blender or food processor and blend until smooth and creamy.
2. Divide among 2 serving glass cup and enjoy immediately.

Nutrition (per serving): 153 calories, | protein 0g, | carbohydrate 27g, | fiber 4g, sugar 4g, | fat 4g, | sodium 0mg | Potassium: 0mg |

Cranberry Banana Smoothie

This recipe is satisfying, easy to prepare and yummy.
Total time: 10 minutes
Prep time: 5 minutes
Cook time: 0 minutes
Servings: 2
Ingredients:
1 cup unsweetened almond milk
1 cup frozen cranberries
1 banana, peel and slice
1 Tbsp. maple syrup
1/2 cup ice cubes
Instructions:
1. Combine all the ingredients in a bowl of a blender and blend until smooth and frothy.
2. Remove from blender and transfer to a serving glass cup. Enjoy!
Nutrition (per serving): 125 calories, | protein 1g, | carbohydrate 27g, | fiber 4g, sugar 15.5g, | fat 1.5g, | sodium 0mg | Potassium: 0mg |

Apple Crisp Smoothie

This recipe is loaded with nutrients and taste so good.
Total time: 10 minutes
Prep time: 5 minutes
Cook time: 0 minutes
Servings: 2
Ingredients:
1/2 cup 2% vanilla Greek yogurt
1/4 tsp. cinnamon
1 cup apple cider
1/4 cup rolled oats
2 Tbsp. pecans
1 cup ice cubes
1/4 tsp. nutmeg
1 cup ice cubes
Instructions:
1. Combine all the ingredients in a bowl of a blender and pulse until smooth and creamy.
2. Transfer smoothie in a serving glass cup and enjoy!
Note: Save the left over in the fridge and try to use within a week
Nutrition (per serving): 232calories, | protein 14 g, | carbohydrate 49g, | fiber 4g, sugar3 2g, | fat 0g, | sodium 0mg | Potassium: 0mg |

Banana Honey Smoothie

Total time: 10 minutes
Prep time: 5 minutes
Cook time: 0 minutes
Servings: 2
Ingredients:
1 banana, peel and sliced
1 tbsp. honey
3/4 cup vanilla yogurt
Instructions:
1. Combine the 3 ingredients in a bowl of a blender and blend until creamy and smooth.
2. Transfer to a serving glass cup and serve immediately.
Nutrition (per serving): 157 calories, | protein 5g, | carbohydrate 35g, | fiber 1.5g, sugar 28g, | fat 1g, | sodium 0mg | Potassium: 0mg |

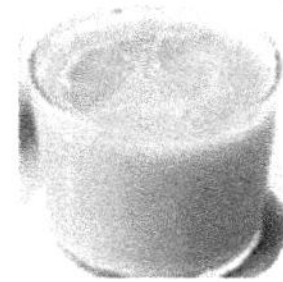

Quick Orange Smoothie

This recipe help you to cool down after workout, it is quick and easy to prepare
Total time: 10 minutes
Prep time: 5 minutes
Cook time: 0 minutes
Servings: 2
Ingredients:
1/4 cup fat-free yogurt
1 navel orange, peeled
1/4 tsp. vanilla extract
2 tbsp. frozen orange juice concentrate
4 ice cubes
Instructions:
1. Combine all the ingredients in a blender or food processor and process until smoothie is smooth and creamy.
2. Transfer to a serving glass cup and enjoy.
Nutrition (per serving): 160 calories, | protein 3g, | carbohydrate 36g, | fiber 3g, sugar 28g, | fat 1g, | sodium 0mg | Potassium: 0mg |

Blueberry and Green Tea Smoothie

This recipe is packed with nutrients and yummy.

Total time: 10 minutes
Prep time: 5 minutes
Cook time: 0 minutes
Servings: 2
Ingredients:
1 green tea bag
1 1/2 cups frozen blueberries
3 Tbsp. of water
2 tsp. honey until it dissolves
1/2 medium banana
3/4 cup calcium fortified light vanilla soy milk
Instructions:
1. In a medium bowl, add 3 tbsp. of water, place in the microwave and let it heat for a while.
2. Add the green tea bag in the hot water for 3 minutes. Remove the tea bags.
3. Add the honey and stir until well mixed.
4. Combine the blueberries, banana and soy milk in a blender and blend until smooth.
5. Add the tea to the blender and blend until creamy.
6. Transfer to a serving cup and enjoy.
Nutrition (per serving): 269 calories, | protein 3.5g, | carbohydrate 63g, | fiber 8g, sugar 38.5g, | fat 2.5g, | sodium 0mg | Potassium: 0mg |

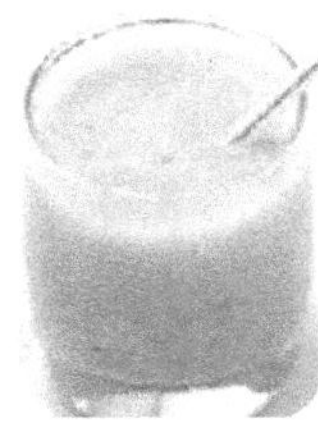

Walnut and banana Shake

This recipe is packed with protein. It makes a good breakfast and I know you love it
Total time: 10 minutes
Prep time: 5 minutes
Cook time: 0 minutes
Servings: 2
Ingredients:
1/4 cup walnuts
1 large frozen banana, cut into chunks
1 tbsp. sugar free cocoa powder
1 cup ice cubes

6 tbsp. chocolate protein powder

1 1/2 cup black coffee

Instructions:

1. Combine all the ingredients in the bowl of a blender and blend until smooth.

2. Divide the smoothie among 2 serving glass cup and serve.

Nutrition (per serving): 264 calories, | protein 24g, | carbohydrate 11g, | fiber 4g, sugar 0g, | fat 11g, | sodium 0mg | Potassium: 0mg |

Papaya and flaxseed Smoothie

This recipe is so yummy and satisfying

Total time: 10 minutes

Prep time: 5 minutes

Cook time: 0 minutes

Servings: 2

Ingredients:

1 tsp. ground flaxseed

1 tsp. coconut extract

1/2 cup crushed ice

1/2 cup fresh pineapple chunks

1 cup of fat-free, plain yogurt

1/2 cup crushed ice

Instructions:

1. Combine all the ingredients in a bowl of a blender and process until smooth and frosty.

2. Transfer smoothie in a serving glass cup.

Nutrition (per serving): 299calories, | protein 13g, | carbohydrate 64g, | fiber 7g, sugar 44g, | fat 1.5g, | sodium 0mg | Potassium: 0mg |

Banana and Almond Smoothie

This recipe is satisfying and keeps you refreshed after and tough workout.

Total time: 10 minutes

Prep time: 5 minutes

Cook time: 0 minutes

Servings: 2

Ingredients:

1/2 cup plain Greek yogurt

1/2 cup coconut water

1 scoop whey protein powder

1 tbsp. hemp seeds

3 tbsp. almond butter

1 cup ice

1 frozen banana, peel and sliced.

Instructions:

1. Combine all the ingredients in a bowl of a blender and blend until smooth and creamy.

2. Divide the smooth is among 2 serving glass cup and serve immediately.

Nutrition (per serving): 329 calories, | protein 17g, | carbohydrate 26g, | fiber 5g, sugar 15g, | fat 17g, | sodium 0mg | Potassium: 0mg |

Watermelon Wonder Smoothie

This is very easy and quick to prepare.

Total time: 10 minutes

Prep time: 5 minutes

Cook time: 0 minutes

Servings: 2

Ingredients:

2 cups of chopped watermelon

1/4 cup almond milk

2 cups ice cube

Instructions:

1. Combine the almond milk, watermelon and ice cube in a bowl of a blender and blend until smooth and creamy.

2. Transfer to a serving glass cup and enjoy.

Nutrition (per serving): 56calories, | protein 2g, | carbohydrate 13g, | fiber 0.5g, sugar 11g, | fat 0g, | sodium 0mg | Potassium: 0mg |

Mixed berries Smoothie

This recipe is energy booster.

Total time: 10 minutes

Prep time: 5 minutes

Cook time: 0 minutes

Servings: 2

Ingredients:

1 cup blueberries

1 1/2 cups chopped strawberries

1 tsp. kale

1/2 cup raspberries

2 Tbsp. honey

1/2 cup ice cubes

1 tsp. fresh lemon juice

Instructions:

1. Combine all the ingredients in a bowl of a blender or food process and blend until smooth and creamy.

2. Transfer smooth to a serving glass cup and enjoy.
Nutrition (per serving): 162 calories, | protein 2g, | carbohydrate 41.5g, | fiber 6g, sugar 32g, | fat 1g, | sodium 0mg | Potassium: 0mg |

Peach and Apricot Smoothie

This recipe satisfying and yummy
Total time: 10 minutes
Prep time: 5 minutes
Cook time: 0 minutes
Servings: 4
Ingredients:
1 apricot nectar, chilled
1 banana
1 container of low-fat peach yogurt
1/2 cup chilled club soda
1 tbsp. frozen lemonade concentrates
Instructions:
1. Combine all the ingredients a bowl of a blender and blend until smooth.
2. Divide smoothie among 4 serving glass cup and enjoy.
Nutrition (per serving): 130calories, | protein 2.5g, | carbohydrate 29g, | fiber 1.5g, sugar 16g, | fat 0.5g, | sodium 0mg | Potassium: 0mg |

Tutti-Frutti Smoothie

This recipe is healthy and refreshing.
Total time: 10 minutes
Prep time: 5 minutes
Cook time: 0 minutes
Servings: 4
Ingredients:
1/2 cup canned crush pineapple in juice
1/2 cup mixed frozen berries
1/2 cup plain yogurt
1/2 cup orange juice
1/2 cup sliced ripe banana
Instructions:
1. Combine all the ingredients in a bowl of a blender or food processor and blend until smooth.
2. Transfer to a serving glass cup and serve.
Nutrition (per serving): 140 calories, | protein 3.5g, | carbohydrate 29g, | fiber 2.5g, sugar 15g, | fat 0.5g, | sodium 154mg | Potassium: 0mg |

Mango and Banana Smoothie

Make this mango and banana smoothie in less than 10 minutes. So yummy!
Total time: 10 minutes
Prep time: 5 minutes
Cook time: 0 minutes
Servings: 4
Ingredients:
1 can of juice-packed pineapple chunks
1 large mango
1 cup fat-free frozen vanilla yogurt
1 ripe banana
4 cup of ice cube
Instructions:
1. Combine all the ingredients in a bowl of a blender or food processor and blend for 1 minute
2. Slowly add the ice cube and blend until creamy and frosty.
3. Divide smoothie among 2 serving glass cup and enjoy!
Nutrition (per serving): 251 calories, | protein 6.5g, | carbohydrate 60g, | fiber 4g, sugar 50g, | fat 0g, | sodium 0mg | Potassium: 0mg |

Peanut butter and mixed berry smoothie

Total time: 5 minutes
Prep time: 5 minutes
Cook time: 0 minutes
Servings: 2
Ingredients:
1 cup frozen mixed berries
1 1/2 cups almond milk or coconut milk
2 tbsp. peanut butter powder
1 scoop dairy free vanilla protein powder
Instructions:
1. Combine all the ingredients in a bowl of a blender or food processor and blend until smooth and creamy
2. Divide smoothie among 2 serving glass cups and serve immediately.
Nutrition (per serving): 140 calories, | protein 21g, | carbohydrate 4g, | fiber 5.0g, sugar 5.0g, | fat 4g, | sodium 0mg | Potassium: 0mg |

Pumpkin Coconut Smoothie

This smoothie is Dairy free and it is very easy to prepare.
Total time: 5 minutes
Prep time: 5 minutes

Cook time: 0 minutes
Servings: 2
Ingredients:
1 frozen banana sliced
1/4 cup organic pumpkin puree
2 tsp. pumpkin pie spice
1 cup almond milk
1 cup ice cube
Instructions:
1. Combine all the ingredients in a bowl of a blender or food processor and blend until smooth.
2. Divide smoothie among serving glass cup and enjoy!
Nutrition (per serving): 292calories, | protein 3g, | carbohydrate 20g, | fiber 2g, sugar 5g, | fat 24g, | sodium 18mg | Potassium: 0mg |

Banana and Chia Seeds Smoothie

This smoothie recipe will keep you refreshing and satisfying for almost the whole day.
Total time: 5 minutes
Prep time: 5 minutes
Cook time: 0 minutes
Servings: 1
Ingredients:
1 banana, peel and sliced
1 cup spinach leaves
1 tbsp. chia seeds
1 cup unsweetened almond milk
1 cup frozen pineapple chunks
Instructions:
1. Combine all the ingredients in the bowl of a blender or food processor and blend until smooth and creamy
2. Transfer smoothie in a serving glass cup and enjoy.

Caramel apple oatmeal smoothie

This recipe is packed with nutrients and it will keep you refreshing
Total time: 3 hour 5 minutes
Prep time: 5 minutes
Cook time: 0 minutes
Servings: 1
Ingredients:
1 cup unsweetened vanilla almond milk
1/2 cup rolled oats
1/2 tsp. ground cinnamon

1 medium apple, peeled and cored
1 tbsp. chia seeds
2 Medjool dates, pitted
Instructions:
1. Combine all the ingredients in a bowl of a blender, mix well, cover and place in the fridge for 3 hours, you can also make it overnight if possible.
2. Remove from fridge and blend until smooth and creamy
3. Transfer to a serving glass cup, add any toppings of choice and enjoy.

Carrot Cake Smoothie

This smoothie is healthy and it taste like carrot cake
Total time: 3 hour 5 minutes
Prep time: 5 minutes
Cook time: 0 minutes
Servings: 1
Ingredients:
1 cup chopped carrots, steamed and cooled
1/2 cup frozen sliced banana
1/4 cup frozen diced pineapple
1/2 cup plain Greek yogurt
1/2 cup unsweetened vanilla almond milk
2 tbsp. toasted walnuts
Pinch nutmeg
1/4 tsp. cinnamon
For topping:
Crushed walnuts
Shredded carrots coconut,
Instructions:
1. Combine all the ingredients in a bowl of a blender or food processor and blend until smooth and creamy.
2. Transfer smoothie in a serving glass cup, add toppings and enjoy.

Cranberry Citrus Smoothie

Total time: 5 minutes
Prep time: 5 minutes
Cook time: 0 minutes
Servings: 1
Ingredients:
3 oranges peeled
1/2 banana frozen
1/2 cup cranberries
1/4 cup Plain Greek yogurt

Cranberry Citrus Smoothie
1/2 tsp. vanilla extract
Instructions:
1. Combine all the ingredients in a bowl of a blender or food processor and blend until smooth and creamy.
2. Transfer smoothie in a serving glass cup, add topping of choice and enjoy

APPITIZER RECIPES

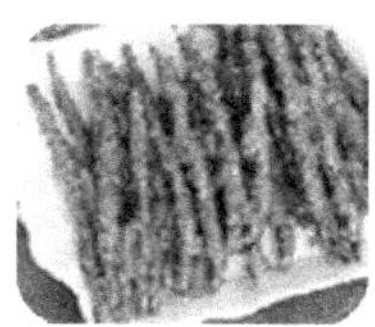

Crunchy oven Baked Green Bean

This healthy appetizer is baked in the oven and it is very easy and quick to prepare. This recipe can also serve as a dinner when you add any veggie of choice to it.
Total time: 25 minutes
Prep time: 10 minutes
Cook time: 15 minutes
Servings: 2
Ingredients:
1 tbsp. all-purpose flour
2 cups fresh green beans, washed and both end trimmed off
1 large egg
3/4 cup panko bread crumbs
3 tbsp. grated parmesan cheese
1/2 tsp. sea salt
Instructions:
1. Preheat the oven to 425°F
2. Place the flour in a bowl and toss the green beans until to lightly coat.
3. Mix panko bread crumbs with parmesan and season with salt
4. Crack the egg in a shallow baking dish and whisk well.
5. Dip the coated green beans in the egg and coat with panko bread crumb and parmesan mixture
5. Spray a baking dish with non-sticky cooking spray. Line the coated green beans in a single layer in a baking dish.

6. Place in the oven and bake until the coating turns golden brown, for about 12 minutes

7. Remove from the oven and serve immediately

Nutrition (per serving): 277calories, | protein 13.9g, | carbohydrate 40.6g, | fiber 4.8g, sugar 6g, | fat 6.8g, | sodium 1047mg | Potassium: 0mg |

Crab Artichoke Toasts

Total time: 35 minutes

Prep time: 20 minutes

Cook time: 15 minutes

Servings: 24

Ingredients:

1 (whole-wheat baguette cut into 24 (1/4-inch-thick) slices

1/2 cup plain nonfat Greek yogurt

3 tbsp. finely chopped fresh flat-leaf parsley divided

1 tsp. fresh lemon zest

1/2 cup gruyere cheese shredded

1 tsp. Fresh lemon juice

1/4 tsp. garlic powder

1 can artichoke hearts drained, patted dry, and roughly chopped

1 can lump crab meat drained

1/4 cup Parmesan cheese finely grated

1/8 tsp. Cayenne pepper

1/4 tsp. kosher salt

1/4 tsp. Black pepper

Instructions:

1. Put the oven rack in the upper third of the oven and set the oven broiler to high. Place a parchment paper in a baking sheet.

2. Arrange the baguette in a single layer in the baking sheet

3. Combine the 2 tbsp. of parsley, Greek yogurt, lemon juice, lemon zest, garlic powder, cayenne salt and pepper together in a large bowl. Add parmesan and gruyere to the bowl and stir well. Gently add the crab and artichokes to the bowl. Taste and make any necessary adjustment.

4. Scoop 1 tbsp. of crab-artichoke mixture on each baguette slice. Place in the oven to broil for 3 minutes or until cheese start to melt. Keep an eye on it to avoid burning.

5. Remove from heat and sprinkle with the remaining 1 tbsp. of parsley. Serve immediately.

Nutrition (per serving): 68calories, | protein 5g, | carbohydrate 9g, | fiber 1g, sugar 0g, | fat 2g, | sodium 0mg | Potassium: 0mg |

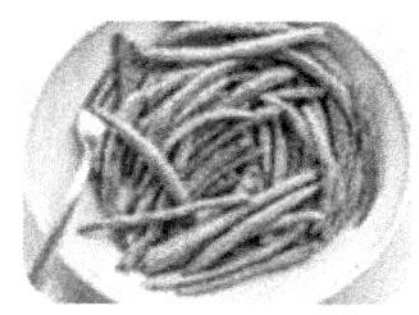

Easy Skillet Spanakopita

Total time: 1 hour
Prep time: 15 minutes
Cook time: 45 minutes
Servings: 4
Ingredients:
4 tbsp. unsalted butter
3 large eggs
1 small onion, diced
 1/4 cup crumbled feta cheese
20 oz. frozen chopped spinach, defrosted and squeeze out the water
1 cup ricotta cheese
2 tsp. dried dill
1 tsp. salt
1/4 tsp. freshly ground black pepper
5 sheets frozen phyllo dough, defrosted
Instructions:
1. Preheat the oven to 375°F
2. Melt 2 tbsp. of butter in a large skillet over medium-high heat, add onion and cook for 5 minute or until softened. Remove from heat and it let cool.
3. Combine the spinach, feta, ricotta, dill, eggs, salt and pepper together in a large bowl and stir well. Add the cooked onion and the dripping from the skillet and stir well.
4. Transfer the mixture from the bowl to the skillet.
5. Melt the remaining butter in a small saucepan and keep a small pastry brush ready.
6. Layer one sheet of phyllo dough over the spinach mixture in the skillet and make sure you cover the rest of the dough to avoid drying out. Use the pastry brush to brush the layer with butter.
7. Layer another sheet of phyllo in opposite direction to properly cover the spinach and brush with butter.
8. Crumble the last 3 phyllo sheet on the top of the skillet and drizzle the rest of the butter on top
9. Place in the oven and bake for 45 minutes or until the dough is golden brown crunchy. Remove from heat and serve immediately.

Nutrition (per serving): 275 calories, | protein 14g, | carbohydrate 20g, | fiber 3g, sugar 1g, | fat 16 g, | sodium 68mg | Potassium: 0mg |

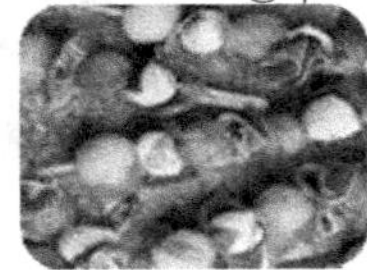

2 Melon Bites Mediterranean Appetizer

This recipe is healthy and very easy to make
Total time: 15 minutes
Prep time: 15 minutes
Cook time: 0 minutes
Servings: 12
Ingredients:
 1/2 honeydew melon, peeled and remove seeds
 24 pistachio nuts, shelled
 6 fresh dates, pitted, cut in half across
 12 toothpicks
 1/2 cup ouzo
Instructions:
1. Use any leftover melon and cut 24 half inch
2. Put the melon cubes in a medium Ziploc bag and add in the ouzo and let it marinate for 2 hours.
3. Drain the ouzo into a glass cup and then thread the melon on the toothpicks
4. Place a cube of the melon on a toothpick add a piece of date and place in another melon cube.
5. Place in the fridge until time of serving. Enjoy!
Nutrition (per serving): 2843.2 calories, | protein 29.3g, | carbohydrate 121.3g, | fiber 71.5g, sugar 49.7g, | fat 268g, | sodium 190.2mg | Potassium: 0mg |

Broccoli Shallots with lemon & Garlic

This recipe is quick to prepare and taste so good; it's a perfect option for busy people.
Total time: 10 minutes
Prep time: 5 minutes
Cook time: 5 minutes
Servings: 4
Ingredients:
1 tbsp. olive oil
1 bunch broccoli, cut into florets
1 shallot, sliced
2 cloves garlic finely chopped

1/4 cup water
Lemon wedges
Sea salt to taste
Freshly ground pepper to taste
Instructions:
1. In a saucepan over medium heat, heat oil. Add the shallots and garlic and cook for a minutes, stir often.
2. Add the broccoli and water, cover the pan and cook until softened for about 4 minutes
3. Remove pan from heat and season with salt and pepper to taste. Serve immediately with lemon wedges.
Nutrition (per serving): 137calories, | protein 6g, |carbohydrate 24g, | fiber 0g, sugar 0g, |fat 4g, | sodium 0mg | Potassium: 0mg |

Avocado Pickles

Total time: 3 hours 15 minutes
Prep time: 5 minutes
Cook time: 10 minutes
Servings: 4
Ingredients:
1 cup distilled white vinegar
1 cup water
1/3 cup sugar
1 clove garlic, thinly sliced
5 sprigs cilantro
1 tbsp. kosher salt
1 tsp. crushed red pepper flakes
2 under ripe avocados, peeled & finely sliced
Instructions:
1. Combine the vinegar, sugar salt and water in a saucepan and place over medium high heat.
2. Bring the mixture to a boil and stir frequently until salt and sugar is totally dissolved. Remove from heat and let it cool.
3. Combine the red pepper flakes, avocado, garlic and cilantro in a mason jar.
4. Pour the cooled mixture into the jar and seal the jar well with a lid.
5. Put the avocado pickles in the fridge for 3 hours or more before serving. Enjoy!

Tomato Mozza Appetizers

Total time: 40 minutes
Prep time: 10 minutes

Cook time: 10 minutes
Servings: 20
Ingredients:
1/2 liters tomato juice
2 grams agar
1/2 mozzarella balls
A drop of vegetable oil
Coarse salt
Instructions:
1. In a medium saucepan, pour the tomato juice and bring to a boil for about 30 seconds
2. Remove from heat and transfer to a flexible molds and put in the fridge for 2 hours.
3. Remove from fridge and unmold into a spoon, add the mozzarella, oil and salt. Enjoy
Nutrition (per serving): 15 calories, | protein 0g, | carbohydrate 1g, | fiber 0g, sugar 0g, | fat 1g, | sodium 40mg | Potassium: 0mg |

Cheesy Bacon Appetizers on Rye

Total time: 28 minutes
Prep time: 10 minutes
Cook time: 10 minutes
Servings: 27
Ingredients:
1/4 cup Jif Extra Crunchy Peanut Butter
1 Ib. Bacon, cooked, drained and crumbles
1 cup mayonnaise
2 tsp. Worcestershire sauce
4 green onions, finely sliced
2 cups shredded cheddar cheese
12 oz. rye bread, sliced party
1/4 tsp. paprika
Instructions:
1. Preheat the oven to 400°F
2. Combine the bacon, peanut butter, Worcestershire sauce, mayonnaise, green onion paprika, and cheese in a medium bowl and mix gently.
3. Assemble the cocktail rye on a baking dish and spread 1 heaping of tbsp. Of bacon mixture each rye square and make sure you spread to edges of the baking dish.
4. Place in the baking dish in the oven and bake for 8 minutes.
5. Remove from the oven and serve immediately.

Nutrition (per serving): 250 calories, | protein 12g, |carbohydrate 8g, | fiber 1g, sugar 0g, |fat 20g, | sodium 630mg |Potassium: 0mg |

Shrimp Appetizers - Easy Party Appetizers

This recipe is so tasty and packed with flavor
Total time: 28 minutes
Prep time: 10 minutes
Cook time: 5 minutes
Servings: 23
Ingredients:
1 avocado, Peel and cut
1/2 cup onion, minced
1/2 lemon juice
1/4 cup coriander
1/2 tsp. salt
250 g cooked shrimp, about 23 shrimps
3/4 tsp. Cumin
1/4 tsp. salt
1/4 tsp. ground black pepper
1 cucumber slice into ½ inch
100 g smoked salmon, slice into 3 inches long and 2 inches wide.
Instructions:
1. Place the cooked shrimp in a bowl add cumin, salt and pepper and set aside.
2. Combine the slice avocado, coriander, lemon juice, onion and salt in a blender and blend until thick and smooth.
3. On a serving plate, assemble the cucumber slices and top with a smoked salmon slice, add 1 tsp. Of guacamole, top with 1 shrimp and then poke 1 toothpick in the centre of the plate. Enjoy!

Nutrition (per serving): 33 calories, | protein 3g, |carbohydrate 1g, | fiber 2g, sugar 1g, |fat 1g, | sodium 196mg |Potassium: 82mg |

Spiced Zucchini

Total time: 60 minutes
Prep time: 30 minutes
Cook time: 30 minutes
Servings: 3 dozen
Ingredients:
4 small zucchini, thinly sliced
1 cup baking mix
1/2 cup thinly chopped onion
3/4 cup grated parmesan cheese, keep 1/4 cup for sprinkling on top

2 Tbsp. lemon thyme finely chopped
2 Tbsp. marjoram, thinly chopped
2 Tbsp. parsley, finely chopped
2 Tbsp. oregano, finely chopped
1 garlic clove, minced
4 eggs, beaten
1/2 cup extra virgin olive oil
Non-Stick Cooking Spray
1/2 tsp. salt
1/4 tsp. pepper

Instructions:
1. Preheat oven to 350°F.
2. Spray a large non- stick pan with a non-sticking cooking spray.
3. Combine all the ingredients in a large bowl and mix well.
4. Transfer to the prepared pan and spread evenly and then sprinkle 1/4 cup reserved parmesan cheese on top evenly.
5. Place in the oven and bake for about 30 minutes or until golden brown.
6. Remove from the oven and let cool a bit before cutting into 4 inches x 2 inches rectangles
7. Serve immediately. Enjoy!

Nutrition (per serving): 60 calories, | protein 2g, | carbohydrate 3g, | fiber 0g, sugar 0g, | fat 4.5g, | sodium 155mg | Potassium: 0mg |

Muffaletta Salad

Total time: 20 minutes
Prep time: 20 minutes
Cook time: 0 minutes
Servings: 16

Ingredients:
1/4 lb. capicola ham, dice
1/4 lb. genoa salami, dice
Grissini bread sticks break in halves
1/4 lb. mortadella, dice
6 oz provolone
1/2 cup olive salad

Instructions:
1. Combine the diced meat, set aside and the dice cheese.
2. In a shot glass, spoon 1 tbsp. of the meat mixture and top with 1 tbsp. of diced cheese and then add 1 tsp. of olive salad mixture.
3. Stick both halves of the grissini breadstick into glass and then serves with a fork or a small spoon.

Nutrition (per serving): 400 calories, | protein 25g, | carbohydrate 10g, | fiber 1g, sugar 0g, | fat28 g, | sodium 1480mg | Potassium: 0mg |

Strawberry Bruschetta

This appetizer is perfect for any occasion, it's quick and easy to prepare.
Total time: 8 minutes
Prep time: 5 minutes
Cook time: 3 minutes
Servings: 16
Ingredients:
1/4 cup Raspberry Balsamic Vinegar
French baguette sliced into 2-3 inch pieces
1 pint strawberries hulled and sliced
Instructions:
1. Place the baguette on a cookie sheet and broil on high for 3 minutes, make sure you check it from time to time to avoid burning.
2. While the baguette is broiling, place the strawberries in a medium bowl and add the raspberry balsamic vinegar and mix well.
3. Top the baguette on the strawberries. Enjoy!
Nutrition (per serving): 100 calories, | protein 3g, | carbohydrate 21g, | fiber 2g, sugar 0g, | fat 0g, | sodium 135mg | Potassium: 0mg |

The End

www.ingramcontent.com/pod-product-compliance
Lightning Source LLC
Chambersburg PA
CBHW070950250726
48663CB00002B/162